Praise for Coping with Menopause

This book provides a comprehensive, practical and humorous guide to navigating menopause. Spanning a diverse range of topics, including the physical, psychological and societal impact, Dr Islam provides positive summaries at the end of each chapter, enabling women to move forward by offering invaluable insights and strategies. Considering the research and theoretical understanding of menopause, she applies her unique and personal perspective using case examples and clinical anecdotes. She is not only an experienced Clinical Psychologist but also a British South Asian who presents the lessons that can be learnt from both Eastern and Western perspectives on menopause. A must read!

Aimee Spector, Professor of Clinical Psychology of Ageing
Director, Menopause Mind Lab, University College London

Low mood, anxiety and depression are common menopause symptoms, and we need a toolkit to help us deal with them. This book offers just that – practical help delivered in a compassionate way.

Fiona Clark, Founder, Menopause Research and Education Fund

Dr Islam's book Coping with Menopause *is an open and honest account of a menopause journey. Menopause has become 'a growing area of interest', in Dr Islam's words, with women becoming more open to discussing menopause and hence they want to learn more.*

Women experience symptoms that can impact mental health, work, social functioning, emotional wellbeing and relationships. The way Dr Islam writes this book is beautiful, empowering women and providing insight into managing common symptoms. This book is a journey that many women will recognise, as Dr Islam opens up about her personal journey in a way that is inspiring and thought-provoking, making readers feel that they are not alone.

I would recommend this book to healthcare professionals and women experiencing perimenopause or menopause. There are so many resources and insights that I, for one, will be recommending others to read. Thank you, Dr Islam, for writing this book.

Teena Mackenzie, Education and Development Lead
British Dermatological Nursing Group

This is a great book which interweaves personal experience with professional expertise and illustrates how a wealth of psychological strategies can be used to manage the day-to-day experience of going through the menopause.

Jane Ogden, Professor in Health Psychology
University of Surrey

This book will be a useful addition to your menopause library, particularly if you are experiencing psychological or cognitive symptoms, and you would like to learn some useful self-help techniques, to improve your quality of life, throughout the menopause transition and beyond.

Diane Danzebrink, Author of Making Menopause Matter and founder of Menopause Support

Coping With Menopause

Coping With Menopause

Psychological tools for navigating the transition and living a balanced life

Dr Momotaj Gafur Islam

SEQUOIA
BOOKS

First published in 2024 by Sequoia Books

ISBN
Print: 9781914110429
EPUB: 9781914110436

A CIP record for this book is available from the British Library

Library of Congress Cataloguing-In-Publication Data

Name: Momotaj Gafur Islam
Title: Coping With Menopause
Description: 1st Edition, Sequoia Books UK 2024
Print: 9781914110429
EPUB: 9781914110436

Print and Electronic production managed by Deanta Global

In memory of my late father. A man of his generation would not have given much thought to the topic of menopause. But as an educated and forward-thinking man with a sense of justice, what he gave me was invaluable – he empowered me to enter higher education and nurtured in me a spirit of determination. For that, I am immensely grateful.

And to my daughter, and nieces, I hope you find this book a helpful resource for when you need it.

Contents

List of Figures and Tables xi
Foreword xii
The Unique Perspective xiii
Acknowledgements xiv

Part I: Understanding Menopause 1

1 Introduction 3
2 My Perimenopausal Journey … So Far 15
3 Overview of Treatment Approaches 24
4 Taking a Holistic Approach 32

Part II: Symptoms and Coping Strategies 43

5 Menopause and Mental Health 45
6 Coping with Stress, Anxiety and Worry 55
7 Mood Management 67
8 Maintaining General Wellbeing 76
9 Problem-Solving Strategies 88
10 Vasomotor Symptoms: Hot Flushes and Night Sweats 97
11 Cognitive Difficulties (Brain Fog) 111
12 Weight Gain and Joint Pain 123
13 Poor Sleep and Insomnia 136

Part III: Impacts and Wider Perspectives 149

14 Impacts on Self-Identity and Relationships 151

15 Menopause at Work: Impacts and Adjustments 165

16 Cultural Differences in Experience, Attitude and Coping 175

Part IV: Conclusion 187

17 The Onward Journey 189

Appendix: The TOOLBOX – A Summary of Key Concepts, Strategies and Tools 199

References 213

About the Author 227

List of Figures and Tables

Figures

4.1 Biopsychosocial-Spiritual Model of the Menopause Experience 34
4.2 Mind Map of the Menopause Experience and Coping Solutions 40
6.1 Vicious Cycle of Anxiety 57
6.2 Coping Cycle of Anxiety 58
8.1 Tabe Analogy for a Balanced Life 79
9.1 Vicious Cycle (blank) 93
9.2 Coping Cycle (blank) 94
10.1 Vicious Cycle of Hot Flushes 103
10.2 Coping Cycle of Hot Flushes 104
10.3 Square Breathing 105
13.1 Vicious Cycle for Anxiety Related to Sleep 138

Tables

7.1 Weekly Mood Tracker 70
8.1 Balanced Lifestyle Log 81
9.1 Menopause Symptoms Experience Log 91
12.1 Food and Feelings Diary 129
13.1 Sleep Diary 144

Foreword

Dr Sarah Swan
Coping With... Series Editor
Consultant Clinical Psychologist

When I was diagnosed with breast cancer in 2019, I knew I was going to have to use my skills as a clinical psychologist to help me cope with the distress that this inevitably caused. Early on in my journey, I had the urge to write, as a way of processing my experiences. I immediately thought it had the potential for a book, but never thought this would come to fruition. But with the support of the Association of Clinical Psychologists, Sequoia Publishing, friends, family and colleagues, I committed to writing the book.

I began to realise what a unique position I held: facing a difficult life event that many others face, but with the knowledge and experience of a long career in helping people with their emotional experiences. Suddenly, it dawned on me that there could be any number of difficult or challenging experiences that other clinical psychologists may have faced. And, like me, they would, in all likelihood, have valuable skills to share with others facing the same situation. And so, the idea for the series was born.

It is an honour to launch the series with my book, Coping with Breast Cancer. And it has been my pleasure to support other clinical psychologists with their writing in order to produce a series of books that will help to bring valuable psychological ideas to a wide audience. With the knowledge and skills of the writers, I am confident that this series will benefit many people facing difficult and challenging situations and given them helpful skills to cope.

The Unique Perspective

Dr Penelope Cream
Clinical and Health Psychologist
Director of Operations
ACP-UK

The Association of Clinical Psychologists (ACP-UK) is delighted to be publishing these important *Coping With…* books. In these pages, clinical psychologists have taken the courageous step of sharing how they applied their skills to their own lives, in order to help others facing similar difficulties and challenges.

The profession of clinical psychology spans many types of psychological approaches across all areas of the lifespan and of individual experiences, from physical health to psychological distress and mental illness, as well as cognitive difficulties, family challenges and workplace problems. Clinical psychologists have rigorous training not only in psychological therapies but also in research methods and using evidence-based practice. They draw on these aspects to inform everything they do, including looking after themselves. These books evidence the flexibility and creativity with which we can use and apply our skills, both to help ourselves and others.

It is not often that clinicians share their first-hand experiences of challenging situations and how they have applied what they have learnt in their training and the many years of experience that follow. I feel very proud of my clinical psychology colleagues who have written this series of books not only for everything that they have experienced with courage and insight but for the generosity and openness with which they want to help other people. It is not easy to combine subjective personal experience with an external clinical perspective; yet in these books, they share the breadth of knowledge and training that the profession brings us.

Acknowledgements

I am grateful to the Association of Clinical Psychologists (ACP-UK), and especially to Dr Sarah Swan and Dr Penelope Cream for the opportunity to write my first book. I have found Sarah's feedback on my early drafts and ongoing guidance throughout the whole process extremely helpful. It has also been beneficial to share ideas and apprehensions with my fellow authors in this series, and I wish them all well with their books.

Being a therapist is a privilege – you are invited into the vulnerable, private space of someone else's world and have the honour of helping them acknowledge and overcome their difficult issues. I hope I have served my clients well over the years. But it is not one-way giving – as a therapist, I have learnt so much from my clients and have shared many a moment of warm connection and laughter too. And of course, I cannot forget all that I have learnt from my educators and colleagues along the way.

I want to thank my friends for their presence in my life. Menopause may have been quite a miserable journey without them. Their encouragement to write a book they are looking forward to reading kept me going whenever I felt a bit stuck. I cannot list all your names, but a special mention to Sidrah and Che for this.

I want to thank my family for their support and for tolerating me not being as available as I might have been at times in the months coming up to completing this project. In particular, I want to acknowledge my son, Siddiq, for being with me on this writing journey – when he was home from university and even when he was away – for being my sounding board during the writing process itself, and for doing the illustrations for each chapter. He listened patiently while I talked about menopause, a fair exchange for me listening about mathematics, I think. I believe he must be the most educated young man on menopause in the country!

Finally, taking in the bigger picture, I have mentioned my faith in my writing, and I am forever grateful to Allah for my life, the good people around me and all opportunities.

Part I

Understanding Menopause

1 Introduction

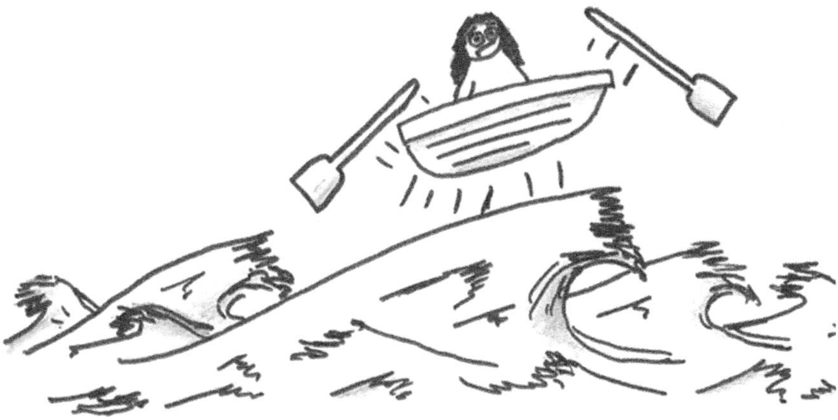

A few introductory facts about menopause

- Menopause is a natural transitional process that every woman* will go through in her lifetime.
- It usually occurs between 45 and 55 years of age. The average age for naturally reaching menopause in the UK, and the Western world generally, is 51.
- An estimated 13 million women in the UK are currently in the menopausal transition – that's a fifth of the population as a whole.
- While 25% are fortunate enough to have little or no symptoms, 75% experience numerous symptoms and find it to be a difficult time to varying degrees.[1]

This book is aimed at helping all women become more informed about the process of menopause and find some potential solutions to make life at this stage more manageable.

*While it is acknowledged that menopause could also be experienced by trans men as well as cisgender women, the terms 'woman' and 'women' are used throughout this book for ease of reference and flow in reading.

About me

I am a 54-year-old woman and a clinical psychologist with 24 years of post-qualification experience. I have been working in the National Health Service (NHS) and other health settings, in academic settings, and more recently in business, all in relation to mental health. I also have lived experience of – and am still living in – the perimenopausal phase for a good number of years. I am looking forward to being on the 'other side' of it (post-menopausal) in the not-too-distant future. I hope that by sharing my personal experience and what I have learnt along the way, I can help you to understand what this phase in life called menopause (peri and post) can look like. I hope to help you feel confident about managing your symptoms and seeking help or treatment where needed, so that you have as smooth an experience of it as possible.

My training as a clinical psychologist included being taught a range of psychological theories and therapeutic approaches, which I had to practise within different clinical settings with a range of client groups. Post-qualification, I have focused mainly on working with adults in secondary care community mental health teams and later in private practice. I have developed my specialty in cognitive behavioural therapy (CBT) and 'third wave' CBT approaches, which I will go on to describe in the upcoming chapters. So, these are the psychological therapeutic approaches I know best. I practise them on myself when needed, as well as with my clients. I will share in this book the strategies that I have found most helpful for managing my perimenopausal symptoms. I will also use my professional skills to draw together knowledge from the existing theory and research literature in this field to discuss recommended coping strategies.

In the spirit of bringing my whole (authentic) self to work, I shall also discuss how my personal and cultural background might have shaped my coping style and perspectives on solutions. I was born in Bangladesh, came to England as a child and grew up in London. I am a married mother of two young adults. I am a practising Muslim, and my spirituality guides me through most things in my life.

Why I wrote this book

I found that I had been suffering perimenopausal symptoms for quite some time, years in fact, before realising what was happening. When I first started noticing my symptoms – which I later learnt was 'brain fog' (explained in Chapter 11) – I thought I was developing early-onset dementia. And I recall for some reason not wanting to 'go there' – like it was something I was afraid to admit – which is so unlike me as I tend to be someone who prefers to tackle things head-on rather than bury my head in the sand. But the thought of dementia was too scary even for me. I only heard of the term 'perimenopause' fairly recently. I have since learnt that many others had/have not heard of it either.

Given that menopause is a natural phase in a woman's life, I started thinking, 'How did that happen?'; 'Why did I not know more about it?'; 'How could I not see what was happening to me?'; and 'How have I let myself suffer for so long without asking more questions ...?' I thought there must be other women out there who do not realise they are experiencing perimenopausal symptoms and may feel quite lost in how or where to seek further knowledge and support.

When I told a friend that I had been worried about developing dementia because of my symptoms, she said, 'If that's what you thought as a professional woman in the health field, what hope is there for the rest of us, the lay-person!' So, I started talking about it more openly with friends and colleagues and realised that there was little information being shared openly. I have found even experts on menopause have reported similar initial thoughts to mine. It is as if most women are just expected to quietly 'get on with it'. That was the case for previous generations, but now women expect to be better informed, and given that the symptoms experienced can have such a significant impact on their lives and be endured for many years, education on this topic is necessary.

From a professional perspective, I realised that I was ill-equipped to help my clients when they were struggling to understand the impact of such symptoms on their lives and how to manage them to get on with their day-to-day functioning. If I didn't even see it in myself, it follows that I didn't see it in my clients either and would not have been curious about whether their difficulties might be related to menopause. I lament this ignorance, but of course now I make more enquiries where relevant with my clients and am more prepared to help normalise and validate their experiences and help them explore ways to manage the symptoms more effectively from a practical and psychological perspective.

As a clinical psychologist, I am not implying that menopause is a mental health condition. However, there is no denying that the symptoms experienced by women, in varying degrees, can have a significant impact on their mental health and emotional wellbeing, on their relationships and on their work and social functioning.

It's pleasing to note that menopause is currently a growing area of interest, and there is a thirst for further knowledge and discussion, as seen for example by the positive response to mainstream television programmes such as 'Sex, Mind and the Menopause' presented by Davina McCall[2] in which she referred to her own experience and explored how menopause can affect the mind as well as the body. Maybe it's because I've got selective attention for the topic now, as well as algorithms being applied in reaction to my online searches, but I am constantly seeing social media postings about it, including celebrities and even royalty describing their experiences, and experts in the field promoting menopause care. Hopefully, this will translate into positive changes in clinical and employment settings. There have even been parliamentary debates and legal cases around this, and there also seems to be a boom in the number of books that have been published in recent years. So, it seems to me that at the moment, 'It's raining men-opause!'. And 'Hallelujiah!', I say. Or rather, 'Alhamdulillah!' (Arabic phrase meaning 'praise be to God'), I should say. Given the silence in this area for far too long, the more the merrier. We have a lot of catching up to do in bringing as much awareness to menopause as we have on other health concerns.

I believe this book will be a welcome addition to the existing literature by not only informing women about menopause and recognising symptoms but also giving them a sense of validation and hope. I want to show that although we may seek professional help when needed, there is a lot we can do ourselves to manage the chaos that menopause can create in our lives and feel more in charge of our own journey. In addition, I hope my exploration of how menopause is perceived and managed within different cultures will be inspiring. And for those yet to reach this phase in life, I hope it provides a realistic perspective on what they might expect and how they might manage the symptoms for a more comfortable transition.

Who this book is for

The proposed audience is mainly women who are currently going through the menopausal transition. They may be aged 40+, but they may also be younger because it can occur very early for some, or simply because they want to be informed. It may also be helpful for partners who want to be informed and supportive. In addition, I hope health professionals in a position to support women experiencing menopausal symptoms will find this book useful to think about symptoms to look out for and ideas for coping strategies to suggest.

Content of the book and how you might use it

This book combines my personal story of living through the menopausal transition with my professional status as a practicing clinical psychologist. So, it will contain personal anecdotes of my experiences, as well as how I draw on psychological therapeutic ideas to cope with my symptoms. My aim is to give you a good balance of what the symptoms can look and feel like and some helpful strategies for managing to live with these symptoms.

After introductions – of myself, of menopause in general and of the psychological approaches I shall be drawing upon – I will describe specific symptoms, possible causes for them and suggested evidence-based coping strategies. I will, of course, not be covering the full range of symptoms, but mainly those that I have experienced on my perimenopausal journey and some from other women's experiences. Please note that as I am not medically qualified, I have steered away from some of the more physical symptoms and any medical advice for treatments. Of course, I cannot talk about menopause and not mention hormonal changes and physical symptoms, but to stay within my area of expertise, the focus in this book is very much on direct psychological symptoms and the secondary effects of these and physical symptoms on our emotional and psychological wellbeing.

The chapters on symptoms consist of the following features:

- What is it – description of the symptom
- What causes it – a brief scientific explanation of suggested causes
- My meno moments – some of my personal anecdotes and reflections
- Coping strategies – ways that you might approach the management of the symptom

At the end of each chapter, you will find the following:

- ★ Key Points box – summary of learning points
- My Gratitude Journal box – things I am grateful for at this point (modelling the gratitude practice described in Chapter 7)
- 'Your turn' – space for you to record your key learning points and gratitude items

I will not be telling you how I 'overcame' menopause with my 'amazing coping strategies'. In fact, I have not overcome it. I'm still here right in it! But I am using the tools I describe to manage my symptoms. I did wonder whether I should be writing this book after I have reached postmenopause so that I could tell the tale of how I 'survived' the transition. Well, firstly, it could go on for a good few years yet! There is no defined 'end point' – so how long am I going to wait? Secondly, I thought it would actually be more 'real' if I observe and describe my experience as I go along. I generally find that after I have gone through things, I tend to forget how difficult it was and can be dismissive of how hard I worked to get through. I think the fallibility of our memories and forgetting the full extent of our pain are natural coping strategies in life. Isn't that what helps us give birth more than once!

The point is to find ways to live with it. It is not a disease for which we are seeking a cure, but a transitional phase that we go through. The difference for us, compared to the experience of our mothers and grandmothers, is that now, rather than hiding away in shame and suffering in silence through it, we are acknowledging that it can be a difficult phase for many of us. And, we'd appreciate appropriate treatment and a few tips on how we might have an easier time of it.

I will go on to explore the potential impact of menopause on our sense of identity; on our relationships with partners, family, friends and in professional settings; and in our ability to function in the workplace or other meaningful roles or activities in our lives. And finally, I will discuss a little about how different societies around the world perceive the menopause and how that might impact treatment and coping. The idea behind this is to explore if perhaps there are areas for learning we can take from others.

It is up to you how you decide to use this book. You might read it cover to cover, which would be much appreciated, of course. Or you might just dip into the chapters that look interesting or most relevant for you. If, like me, you are currently going through perimenopause, I would recommend reading the introduction chapter first, and like I have done in Chapter 2, having a think about when it all might have started for you, and which symptoms you might have experienced so far. This may give some perspective on your experience so far, and you might surprise yourself with how you have already been coping . If you are already well informed on the topic but are looking for coping strategies, you might specifically read the sections on the symptoms that you are currently trying to manage.

At times, things may sound very doom and gloom when talking about menopause, especially when we talk about the numerous symptoms that might be experienced. However, it doesn't necessarily have to be so. Once we are informed, we are empowered. We can then take whatever action we feel appropriate for our individual situations and lifestyles. We can feel confident about requesting treatments which might suit us. And we might even have a positive attitude towards this transition period and come out feeling quite rejuvenated as we go forth on our onward journey in life.

In whatever way you choose to use this book, I hope you find it a reassuring and helpful read. I hope my insights will help you to better understand and navigate the choppy waters of menopause and have a smooth journey of it overall.

What is menopause? And what does it look like?

According to historical research on menopause, Aristotle made reference to it saying it occurs at the age of 40.[3] The word menopause is thought to have been coined by a French physician named Charles Pierre Louis De Gardanne in 1821. It is derived from the Greek words *mēn* (month) and *pausis* (pause), hence meaning the 'end of monthly cycles', that is, the ceasing of menstrual periods. I always like to start by defining my terms – to put things into context so that we have a shared understanding of what we are talking about. So, let's get familiar with the language when talking of menopause before we go on to discuss things in more detail.

Menopause: You reach menopause when you have gone through 12 consecutive months without a menstrual period. The operative word here is 'consecutive', as you will see in later discussions. As you age, there is a gradual change in the balance of your body's hormones. Menopause happens when your ovaries are no longer producing sufficient oestrogen, the female sex hormone, to release an egg each month – thus marking the end of your menstrual cycles.

It usually happens between the ages of 45 and 55, with the average age being 51. It can sometimes happen earlier and is referred to as early menopause when it happens before 45. One in 100 women reach menopause before 40 and one in 1000 before 30.[4] When early menopause occurs naturally, it is called premature ovarian insufficiency (POI). Menopause can also be triggered by certain treatments such as chemotherapy or radiotherapy or surgery to remove the ovaries (oophorectomy) or the uterus (hysterectomy). Sometimes it may not be possible to determine what caused an early menopause.

Perimenopause: This is the phase leading up to menopause when you are continuing to have periods but you experience shifts in your menstrual cycle and flow of your periods. You are also likely to experience other symptoms related to the drop in hormone levels. This phase can start years before your menstrual periods finally stop. There is a range of durations reported, but the general consensus is that it can last between 2 and 10 years, with the average being seven years. It is not known what causes this phase to go on so long.

Postmenopause: This is the rest of our life after you have experienced menopause. You can continue having symptoms when you are postmenopausal mainly due to depleted hormone levels. It can take years for your body to settle into your new hormone levels.

So, technically, menopause is reached on the day you have not had a period for 12 months. But you can only know this in hindsight by tracking back to your last period, which can in itself be a difficult task unless you keep stringent records of your menstrual cycle. This is because you can go for months without a period, then boom, you get an unexpected period, and you're back to counting from the start again. Last year, I went six months without a period and then got a surprise one, just as I arrived on the beautiful island of Santorini with my light summer dresses for a much-needed holiday! Then, I went for a stint of eight months and had a one-off heavy bleed. On my current count, I'm into my fifth dry month and hoping to make it to 12, but who knows when Auntie Meno might strike again! I've heard women talk about going 11 months without, then getting a period. It's like running in a race and having a fall, but instead of picking yourself up and carrying on, you are made to go back to the start line. This can make you feel disappointed and cause you to feel anxious about the uncertainties.

As you can see, menopause is not a tidy affair where we just stop bleeding one day and are off on our merry way to middle-aged freedom from the hassle of periods, as I had thought in my ignorance. In fact, it is a process, and the transition from perimenopause (which is even harder to track the start of) to menopause can take a long time. And even more of a shock to my ignorant mind was the news that the symptoms do not necessarily stop at menopause, but can go on for months or years afterwards! The experience will be different for each woman. Some of us might get through it fairly smoothly while barely noticing symptoms, and others of us may find it to be a long and arduous journey.

You may often hear women say they are 'menopausal' or 'going through the menopause'. This could refer to any of the above stages when they are experiencing symptoms. I will use the terms 'menopause' and 'menopausal' to refer to the whole period of transition from peri- to post-menopause and experiencing of symptoms in those phases – mainly because perimenopause and postmenopause are a bit of a 'mouthful', even when reading them in your head!

How do we know if we are going through perimenopause?

If you are under 45 and experiencing what look like menopausal symptoms, you can get a blood test done to check your level of follicle-stimulating hormone (FSH), which is responsible for regulating the oestrogen in your body. For over 45s, there is not really a way of formally diagnosing that you are in perimenopause. It is a gradual process, and there is no single test that can determine if it has started. Technically, you could have the FSH test, but most doctors say that it is not worth doing this because hormone levels fluctuate so much by this age, so it would only be reflecting your hormone levels in that moment of testing and not be a reflection of your hormone levels in general.

Some doctors might do a thyroid function test to rule out other factors because some of the symptoms of an underactive thyroid (hypothyroidism) and menopause are similar and can occur at around the same age. Also, hypothyroidism can increase the risk of long-term complications during menopause, so it can be useful to know this if you are perimenopausal. There are some over-the-counter home testing kits which claim to determine if you are currently into perimenopause or menopause. These are usually blood tests requiring a finger-prick or urine tests which measure FSH levels. They are not considered to be very accurate by medical professionals and not recommended.[5]

So, it is usually down to you to report changes in your menstrual cycle and other symptoms experienced to your doctor, who will consider this in relation to your medical history. Age is, of course, a factor, but many women have reported being dismissed by their GP (general practitioner or primary care physician in the UK) purely on the basis of age, when it is known that symptoms can show up much earlier than the expected age of 45. I found that it can even be ignored when you are over 45. After having visited my GPs with symptoms for years, from when I was about 47 years old, not once did one of them mention the possibility of my symptoms being related to menopause. It was only after I heard the term perimenopause for the first time that I mentioned it to one GP, and there was an unenthusiastic 'yes perhaps', yet still no suggestions for looking further into this.

Further reason for us to educate ourselves on the menopause is that there has historically been minimal training on the menopause at medical school, leaving many doctors not fully informed about the symptoms to look for in their patients, unless they are of the few who have specialised with further training or research. It is encouraging to note that the UK government has introduced a 'Women's Health Strategy' to tackle the 'gender health gap', which will require doctors in training to have mandatory specific teaching and assessment on women's health, including menopause.[6]

What symptoms might we experience during perimenopause and postmenopause?

Throughout the menopausal transition, there are a whole array of symptoms that we may experience. One of the first indicators that we are entering into perimenopause is when we notice changes in the usual pattern of our periods. This is usually due to the levels of hormones, which normally regulate the menstrual cycle – oestrogen and progesterone – fluctuating all over the place. This can lead to irregularity in periods from very frequent periods to missed periods and variations in flow from very light to heavy periods. And these irregularities can go on until the periods stop completely. It can be hard to know when that will be, and we will not actually be sure until our 12th month without a period. There will be advice on tracking symptoms in Chapter 9.

Then, there are a range of other physical symptoms also related to fluctuations in hormone levels, like hot flushes, vaginal dryness and emotional reactions like mood swings. As mentioned above, these symptoms can start long before our periods stop and continue afterwards. It is not the same experience for all women. Some will have few symptoms or have quite a few, but they might be subtle and not cause too much discomfort. For others, their symptoms might be severe, interfere significantly with their daily living and cause much distress. For some, it might last a few months, and for others it may go on for years. Symptoms can not only vary in severity, but they can also change over time. For example, we might have significant hot flushes and night sweats for a few months, and these improve; then, we notice more brain fog moments. Some symptoms, such as joint pain and vaginal dryness, can persist after we stop menstruating when we are in post-menopause. Fortunately for most of us, symptoms tend to settle over time.

Some of the most common symptoms of menopause include the following:

- *Irregular periods* – missed periods or prolonged periods; there may be a change in flow of bleeding with maybe only spotting for a few days to unusually heavy bleeding for a number of days
- *Hot flushes* - suddenly feeling hot, sweaty and flushed, usually in the face, neck and chest. This can be followed by feeling a cold chill which is equally uncomfortable
- *Night sweats* – these are hot flushes that occur at night and can often wake us up and leave us soaking in our nightwear and bedding (Hot flushes and night sweats are jointly referred to as *vasomotor symptoms* because they occur when there are changes in blood vessel activity in the body.)
- *Poor sleep and tiredness* – sleep may be disturbed by being woken by night sweats or anxiety, causing tiredness and irritability. Other factors like physical pains, anxiety, stress, iron deficiency may also cause lack of sleep.
- *Mood shifts and anxiety* – becoming unexpectedly tearful, sad or angry for no apparent reason; the unpredictable nature of some of the symptoms may cause anxiety.
- *Brain fog* – experiencing cognitive problems like lapses in memory, lacking focus and difficulty in concentrating
- *Vaginal discomfort* – reduced oestrogen can cause vaginal tissues to become thinner and drier and make us more prone to pain, itching or discomfort during sex
- *Lower libido* – depleted hormone levels can reduce physical arousal and desire for sex
- *Changes in body shape and weight gain* – this can happen over the time of this transitional phase due to a number of factors
- *Muscle aches and joint pains* – feeling tightness in muscles and stiffness in joints
- *Hair and skin problems* – for example, thinning hair and/or dry itchy skin
- *Severe headaches* – menstrual headaches or migraines may feel more severe during perimenopause

This is not an exhaustive list of the symptoms that women report during their menopausal transition. If you Google 'How many symptoms of menopause are there?', you will get anything from 22 to 48 to 60. Most commonly, there are lists of 34 symptoms of menopause. Having looked at one of these lists, a bit like those lists you get on social media where you tick off how many countries you've travelled to, I'm not boasting but I can say that I have had 20 on my menopausal journey, so far! On a more serious note, there is no scientific evidence to back these figures up. All we know is that there are many symptoms that women may report during this transitional phase.

We need to keep in mind that our menopausal transition is co-occurring with our normal ageing process, and we may also be experiencing other physical conditions or external stressors at the same time. Therefore, we cannot simply attribute all symptoms during this time to menopause. And for our own sake of getting the correct treatment, with the help of our doctor, we need to rule out other potential explanations for symptoms, as menopause may not be the only contributing factor.

How does menopause affect our emotional and mental health?

Although menopause is essentially a biological/chemical process in the body, and it follows that many of the symptoms of menopause look predominately physical in nature, it is not hard to see how the process affects the mind as well as the body. For example, if we regularly experience night sweats, we're likely to wake up at least once or several times and may not be able to get back to sleep easily. This sleep disturbance may make us tired and irritable and affect our concentration during the day. The unpredictable nature of hot flushes can make us anxious when going out, as we don't know when the next one will strike and how we will manage it. Brain fog can also cause anxiety and make us worry about making mistakes or embarrassing ourselves in front of others. Furthermore, menopausal symptoms can have a big impact on our sense of who we are, on our relationships, and on our family life, work and social life.

What can I do to relieve my symptoms?

As mentioned above, the experience of menopause will be different for each woman, and equally in terms of management of symptoms some approaches might work for some and not for others. Fortunately, there are many effective coping strategies and treatment approaches that can be tried. A starting point might be to assess our lifestyle and be equipped with better knowledge of what is going on for us during this transitional phase. We might consider making adjustments in our diet, exercise or sleep routine, for example, to see what impact we might have in reducing our symptoms. Many women report relief from symptoms using hormone replacement therapy (HRT), which is aimed at replacing the lost hormones to help relieve symptoms. Others prefer natural (herbal) remedies or complimentary treatments. Psychologically, there are ways we can put things into perspective and learn strategies for coping and feeling better about ourselves and also seek support from those around us.

Key points

There is a long list of symptoms that women may experience during their menopausal journey

There are many forms of help available to manage symptoms

Knowledge will empower you to find what works for you.

Today I am grateful for:

Being able to educate myself on menopause and how it impacts my life

Finding strategies that work for my mind and body.

The opportunity to share my experience and knowledge

Your turn:

List your **key learning points** from this chapter

List two or three things (big or small) you are **grateful for** right now

2 My Perimenopausal Journey ... So Far

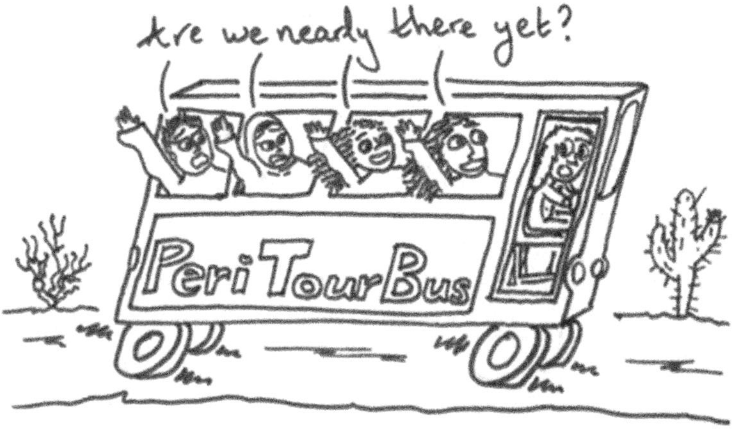

Starting with periods ... Trigger warning: There will be blood!

Most of us will be able to think back and recall when we started our periods, as it is a clear and significant event in our lives. If I do this chronologically, my journey with my womb functioning, as it were, started at the age of 10. Of course, I am not going to chart out all my menstrual cycles since then. The reason I'm referring back to this is because a couple of recent conversations triggered some memories for me that do link to my current circumstances. The first conversation I had was with a colleague of a similar age. Talking about the menopause, we somehow got onto the topic of menstruation and how neither of us had been prepared for the start of our periods. The second conversation was after dinner that day when I was telling my husband about the chat with my colleague in the context of writing this book. I began telling him about when I started my periods – not a topic that has come up before in our 30 years together. While telling the story, I suddenly began to cry and couldn't contain myself. This surprised me. It was then that I realised my experience might be considered an emotional trauma, and these conversations had triggered me.

So, what can be traumatising about starting your periods, a most natural experience? Well, I was 10 years old, which was younger than the average age of 12 years that girls start menstruating,[1] though I understand they can start as young as eight, and research shows that many girls are starting sooner nowadays.[2] I was completely unprepared for it so I didn't know what was happening to me, and not only did I feel I couldn't talk with anyone about it (including my mother), I felt I needed to hide it. We didn't talk about private matters like this. And I was in a house with three males. But I think all that was still within the normal experience of an average Asian girl in the 1980s. I think the traumatising factor was that within the context of this background, I had the heaviest first bleeds that even if I had been prepared for my periods, I could never have imagined. And I still do not think such heavy bleeds at that age were normal. A bit of graphic detail, but all I can say is that I had clots the size of golf balls being emitted from my 10-year-old body. The extent of the bleeding was so bad that I felt that I could not leave the bathroom because as soon as I did, I needed to rush back. Living in a flat with only one bathroom and without anyone else knowing what was going on, others were getting annoyed at me for hogging the bathroom. Meanwhile, I was sitting on the bathroom floor feeling very weak, worrying about what was happening to me. I expected to have bleeding but didn't think it should be this bad. I remember feeling very scared and very alone. And this happened each month for a good while.

So, as you can see, I did not have the best start to this journey. I am very grateful to my body for enabling me to spring forth two beautiful children. But my womb and I have been in a rocky relationship from the start, and my heavy periods in recent years have outdone even those in the early years. Prepare for more blood scenes!

I am fortunate to not have had pre-menstrual syndrome (PMS) symptoms (well, maybe a bit that I'm aware of, but not like I've seen in others I know), but I have always had heavy bleeding which I just got used to and just had to battle through. I recall a number of years ago, when I had particularly heavy bleeding, starting to wonder if they really were normal and visiting my GP to ask. Her response – 'That's just you!' Well, there you go, it was 'just me'. After all, wasn't I the girl who had started with the golf balls! So, I had to suck it up and carry on regardless!

And on we go …

Fast forward over 40 years, and I'm now trying to pinpoint the start of my perimenopausal journey. This is not as easy to do as it is for the start of your periods. That's because you don't know you are at the start of something, and when you do realise you are on this journey, you have to try to trace back and identify when you might have taken that 'first step'. Of course, if I was better informed of this phase called perimenopause, I might have thought to make a note of changes in my periods from when they started.

With hindsight, I think I have traced it back to an incident about seven years ago. I was on one of my heavy periods on a day when I work in private practice. So, I had gone to the clinic prepared with all the usual sanitary paraphernalia. After my last session that afternoon, I popped into the bathroom. While I was on the loo, the floodgates opened! And they just would not 'shut' – I literally could not get off the loo. I had used up my supply of sanitary pads for the day, and I was fast running out of the toilet roll supply in the cubicle. To make matters worse, this was a small clinic with one bathroom – for both men and women to use. I heard one or two people come into the bathroom and leave again when they saw the cubicle occupied. Did this trigger memories of the 10-year-old? I don't know, I was in survival mode in those moments, but at some visceral level, it probably did.

So how was I going to get out of this predicament? Trying not to panic, I thought, 'I just need enough padding to get out of here and get home', which was a 20-minute walk away. Fortunately, because I was leaving the clinic, I had brought my handbag with me into the cubicle. So, I reached for my phone and called home. Another stroke of luck was that my daughter would be home – the one time I was actually pleased with how little in-person teaching time she had at university and was given so much time for 'self-directed learning', considering the tuition fees. I called her and explained the situation, then had to wait while she walked over to the clinic with extra sanitary towels. I had to sit silently on the toilet and let others who needed the bathroom go and complain to reception about it being occupied for so long. It felt like such a long wait, especially as I'd already been there quite some time trying to deal with the bleeding, which had not yet stopped. When my daughter eventually got to me, I put myself together and sneaked out so no-one knew it was me who had been hogging the bathroom! Writing this, I am reminded of the time when I caught the receptionist at the clinic describing me to a colleague as her 'role model'. I didn't feel much like a role model then!

That evening, I was telling my cousin who is only a few years older than me what had happened and she said, 'This is it, it's the beginning of the end!'. She went on to say that it was like having a big 'splurge' before you 'completely dry up'. She didn't use the word menopause, and neither did I think of this word in my head, but somehow, I instantly knew what she meant. I knew she meant my periods were coming to an end, which is what I understood menopause to be. But how did I know? Did I vicariously pick this kind of knowledge up from the women around me? Bangladeshis of a certain age have this habit of talking in roundabout ways. It was since then that I got the idea that menopause was looming, and it was only a matter of time before I just stopped having periods. Little did I know then how much more there was to it than just one day your 'monthly guest' (another Bengali phrase) doesn't show up!

Also, I was about 47 years old and hadn't thought I was anywhere near old enough for menopause. Wasn't it what happened to older women, not those my age who these days were still getting pregnant themselves never mind becoming 'granny age'? Nonetheless, this conversation triggered me to mention the 'M' word to the doctor whom I saw the next day for an emergency appointment to stop my incessant bleeding. He said it was a possibility but didn't seem that interested and prescribed me Norethisterone, then Tranexamic Acid (two drugs used for controlling menstrual blood flow) – these two went on to become my reliable travel buddies on this journey for a few years to come; that is, until they gave up on me and we parted ways – I never found out why they stopped working for me.

Then, about a year later, I was sent for an abdominal scan for some other issue I don't recall and discovered another stumbling block along the road – I had several sizeable fibroids (non-cancerous growths that develop in or around the womb). It was asserted that these, which had developed over a number of years, were what was causing my heavy bleeding. I thought back to the GP who had dismissed my concern about heavy bleeding as 'just you' and felt angry – with her, for not sending me for a scan then, and with myself, for not pushing for further investigation. I spent the next few years going back and forth from appointments between my GP and consultants at numerous hospital departments – diagnostic imaging, gynaecology and gastroenterology – being investigated for problems from my abdomen and below. Being quite an impatient person, I tend to want things done immediately, but when a gastroenterology consultant asked if I had a 'sense of urgency', he put a whole new meaning to it. I somehow felt relieved that he 'knew' my problem at the time, in the gastrointestinal sense!

I had both the male gynaecology consultants and the male gastroenterology consultant advising me to have a hysterectomy so I can be 'done with' all this heavy bleeding and other problems. And I was suffering so much – for example, on one occasion I had a whole month of non-stop heavy bleeding – that I was close to making that decision, but for the fact that I hate any kind of surgery and I didn't like the idea of needing months to recover from it. At the back of my mind was also the thought that my womb is what makes me a woman and I didn't want to lose it. I felt more supported to consider other less drastic options when my female GP said, in response to me reporting what the consultants had advised, 'Well that's easy for them to say, they wouldn't be having a whole chunk of their body removed!'. Of course, for some women, a hysterectomy may become a medical necessity or an informed choice based on their medical history. But in my case, I am thankful for that nod from my GP towards my way of thinking and am pleased to still have my womb.

The point of mentioning all this is that it all distracted me from the idea of menopause for a number of years. The medics were busy looking into all the other possibilities of what was going on and didn't ever mention that anything could be linked to menopause, until I questioned it myself. At this stage, a well-known consultant gynaecologist – whom I had heard of, so was pleased to be seeing – checked my hormone levels and said, 'You are way off menopause'. But, they didn't mention that there is this transition phase called perimenopause. Given I was almost 50 years old at the time, shouldn't they have told me that there is this potentially very long run up to the medical definition of menopause?

Am I developing early onset dementia ...?

During this period of ongoing investigations from my waist down, I started experiencing problems higher up in my anatomy. There was a period of absent-mindedness, forgetfulness and general memory loss that my family were accusing me of. I say 'accusing' because, of course, I was defensive and genuinely did not believe that I had said this or that already, or left this and that on and upon being told this a few times I became annoyed. But then, it was when I noticed it happening outside the home, more specifically at work meetings that I started opening up to the possibility that I was forgetting what I'd said and repeating myself or making mistakes in my speech. I began observing myself more – I felt shocked at what I noticed.

I was a trustee for a charity and I remember getting frustrated at board meetings when words I wanted weren't coming into my head. I noticed one or two looks, as if colleagues were wondering why I was saying something again (maybe I'd just said it earlier) and when I struggled to find words. These observations started to make me anxious about speaking up in meetings. But anyone who knows me knows that I hate not having my say, so then that became frustrating too. I'll discuss how this kind of experience becomes a vicious cycle and how to cope with it in upcoming chapters.

I remember one particular meeting at my university-based job when I had just done a group supervision session with some trainees and immediately afterwards, I attended a supervisors' meeting to discuss the progress of the trainees, and I couldn't remember a couple of their names. It was only six names to remember, and I had been supervising them weekly for months. I kept getting two particular trainees muddled up (they did have similar features!). I remember saying something about being sleep deprived, which was true. To this day, I can see a sort of concerned expression on a colleague's face in that meeting.

I recall that moment as the trigger to my thoughts about developing early onset dementia and the feeling of fear about what I thought was to come. It was around that time that I had watched a film called 'Still Alice' (based on the book by Lisa Genova) with Julianne Moore's excellent performance as Alice, a university professor who starts noticing cognitive problems. There is a moment when Alice is giving a lecture and goes completely blank mid-sentence. I remember fumbling around for words during lectures at times and quickly having to grasp at a simpler alternative word. Alice goes on to be diagnosed with early-onset Alzheimer's disease, and watching her decline, while identifying with her character, felt very scary. I recently watched the film again and noticed that she briefly mentioned that menopause was initially considered to explain her symptoms but dismissed after further investigation. I had not even picked up on this bit in the film at all when I watched it the first time. Menopause just was not on my radar at the time.

But again, I must have got distracted by life, maybe I put it down to stress and sleep problems, and carried on. I suppose that's how we manage to keep going with these symptoms for years, as well as the way the symptoms keep shifting. It was when the symptoms of cognitive difficulties re-surfaced, especially in combination with the sleep deprivation that I became more worried and decided I needed to look into things further, seek help and make the necessary changes. It led me to worry about my functioning at home and at work and consider making changes at work, such as cutting down my hours or leaving altogether.

So, when did I start pinning it down to the menopause?

I think, like for most women, it was the hot flushes that did it! This is probably the symptom we all associate with menopause, and so it's often not until we get this 'obvious' sign that it finally clicks what is going on. For me, I'm not sure if the hot flushes were even that obvious to start with. I could not say when I had my first hot flush. I probably assumed I had a temperature or something the first few times. I ask myself sometimes, exactly how dim was I on this topic! It's not really until a whole gamut of symptoms – brain fog, hot flushes, night sweats, dryness and so on – hit me that I finally twigged I was in the midst of perimenopause. I'll share these delights of the journey with you in the upcoming chapters.

Are we nearly there yet?

So here I am seven years after that first awful moment in the clinic loo which may or may not have been the starting point of my journey. And it's not over yet!

So, what I'm finding so far is that I am working my way through the symptom list. They don't come all at once, thank goodness, but in spates; so I've had episodes of muscle tension, then vaginal dryness, then joint aches, then a period of hot flushes and another period of brain fog, or sometimes a few symptoms together for a while. It's like they take turns to keep you on your toes. You feel like you are constantly in a state of flux, and like this, you can surprisingly tot up quite a few years being perimenopausal and feeling drained from all the shifting symptoms.

'A day in the life' of a perimenopausal working mum

So, what's it like being a working mother living with perimenopausal symptoms on a day-to-day basis? Well, it's hard to describe a typical day, as the symptoms are unpredictable in nature and vary in severity from day to day. So, I'll describe what might happen on a good day and a not so good one. Like many clinical psychologists and women at work in general, I have a variety of tasks that make up 'work'. In a week I see clients for therapy, work as a consultant, have a teaching day, supervision groups, meetings related to my role as trustee of a charity, and so on. And of course, as a working mum, somewhere in there, I need to squeeze in family time and running a home. Then there's this book to write.

What a good day might look like ...

On a good day, I can get by with some of my symptoms bothering me but not to such a great extent that I can't achieve the tasks of the day to a relatively good standard. I'm a lists person, so I have to-do lists everywhere – on my phone, in my diary, on post-it notes – with different categories (e.g., work, home, personal) and various levels of prioritisation. The post-it-note is usually my 'list for the day' – the essential tasks for that day, which I cross off with a sense of satisfaction once completed.

On a good day, I'll have the occasional hot flush, take a moment to let it pass, and if I'm in company, hope no-one has noticed. Recently, a female colleague of similar age noticed me looking flustered, so I whispered, 'hot flush' and she gave me an empathic nod. (As a side note, I just had a brain fog moment writing this – it took me four attempts at trying to spell 'whispered' before it looked right!)

On a good day, I might come away from a meeting having only struggled to find one or two words and not felt embarrassed that others have picked up on this. On a good day, I'll tick off most of my list as done and only transfer one or two items onto a fresh post-it-note and scrunch up the one for that day. And at home, I'll switch off from work mode, get on with whatever needs doing and connect with my family.

Now, let's take a look at a bad day ...

On a bad day, I'll have numerous hot flushes and chills (either following the hot flushes or independently), feel tired from having woken up several times in the night sweating, and find it hard to concentrate or find words. I'll struggle through meetings. These can be especially hard when I am supposed to be the 'expert', for example, in a business pitching meeting and I can't remember the psychological term for something, struggle for a bit and come up with 'x' instead of 'y'.

As a clinical psychologist with a private practice, of course, it is desirable to get telephone or email enquiries about potential new client referrals. But on a bad day, it can make me sigh and want them to go away.

I recall one particularly bad day at work when I had just got through a morning of facilitating two 2-hour group supervision sessions back-to-back, had a half-hour lunchbreak and then had to give a lecture in the afternoon. Feeling really exhausted from sleep deprivation, so not my usual personable self, I arrived to a room full of trainees. The room had no windows and felt a bit stuffy. For the first time ever, I actually gave the lecture mostly sitting on a chair and did not try very hard to engage the students. It was not surprising that this was the first lecture where I did not receive my usual positive student feedback, and one of them actually mentioned my sitting on a chair on their feedback form – more reason to feel awful!

On a day like that, at home I'll be irritable, moan about others not pulling their weight with household chores, and not have the energy to ask how anyone else is doing. And if things are really bad like when I have joint pains in my hands making basic physical tasks like opening jars difficult, I have on occasion ended up frustrated and in tears. I think this can unnerve my family who see me as the 'strong' one and in turn makes me feel like I'm letting them down. On a bad day, I've done well to tick a few items off my post-it-note to-do list, but it's not ready to scrunch up yet..

On writing this book

So, how does one write a book on menopause while actually transitioning through it on this rollercoaster of symptoms? At first it seemed like a great idea. Very soon, doubts started to creep in, especially when my brain fog was at its worst and when I was most fatigued from sleep deprivation caused by night sweats. But then, I convinced myself I can do it. Here are a few snippets from my diary to demonstrate my thinking:

Getting anxious about writing this book.
*I can't even focus on reading a book, how the **** am I supposed to write one!*
I can't concentrate to finish a page without re-reading each paragraph, and I can't remember words I know in order to string a good sentence together.
But what I really hate is the idea of quitting – I'll use all the strategies I know to cope, and I will write this book, insh'Allah! (Arabic term meaning 'God-willing').
Then maybe I can write my second book on 'how to cope with writing a book while going through menopause', haha.

And so, the journey continues. 'Am I really coping?', I sometimes ask myself. Do I not sometimes feel like I'm getting through each day by the skin of my teeth? An obsolete definition for 'coping' is 'to meet in combat' and perimenopause can indeed feel like being in a battle at times. The Merriam-Webster Dictionary definition of coping is 'to deal with and attempt to overcome problems and difficulties'. The fact that I am seven years in and have been overcoming the difficulties by my chosen means indicates that I am coping. On most days I cope well, and other days not so well, but that is understandable on this rollercoaster of a journey. On the whole, I manage to do my work well, run an organised household, maintain relationships and find time for enjoyable activities; so I must be doing something right. I am living with perimenopause and feel physically and mentally well most of the time – and that's good enough for me. I hope, with the benefit of my insights and sharing my strategies, you will cope even better.

Key points

Each menopausal journey is unique

It can be helpful to reflect and chart your symptoms

Symptoms fluctuate - acknowledge the good days and be kind to yourself on the bad days

Today I am grateful for:

Getting through the tough early start

Having realised that I am going through perimenopause when I did

Having many more good days than bad days

Your turn:

List your **key learning points** from this chapter

List two or three things (big or small) you are **grateful for** right now

3 Overview of Treatment Approaches

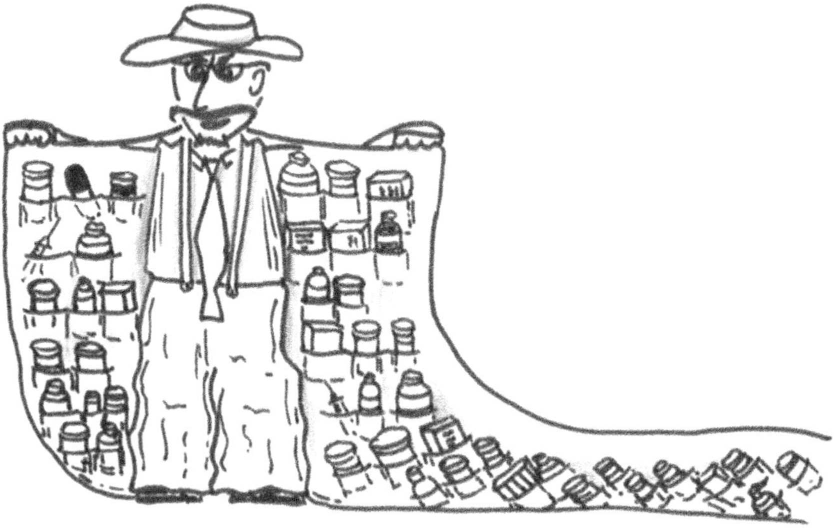

There are many different perspectives on how we approach the management of our menopausal symptoms. Much of this is down to personal choices, and sometimes there may be restrictions on our choices due to our personal medical history. I will briefly describe those formally recommended in government guidelines and simply acknowledge the other types of approaches many women may take. As this book is about my lived experience and my suggested coping strategies from a psychological self-management perspective, these two areas will be my focus. Like many women, I have also tried or considered some non-psychological methods or medical approaches in trying to manage my symptoms. I will describe some of these where relevant, but only anecdotally.

If you are interested in using any of the approaches instead of or in addition to the practical and psychological tools that I describe in this book, you will need to do your own research into them from reliable sources (see resources section at the back for further reading).

Hormone replacement therapy (HRT)

Hormone replacement therapy (HRT) – or menopausal hormone therapy (MHT) as it is sometimes called – refers to the use of synthetic hormones to supplement those lost during the menopausal transition. It is based on the idea that, as many of our menopausal symptoms are thought to be due to a depletion of hormones, if we replace or replenish those hormones, it should bring our hormone levels back up and, in turn, reduce the symptomatic effects related to the depletion of hormones.

The history of HRT makes for interesting reading, as it has been quite controversial. It became available on prescription in the 1960s and was particularly popular by the early 1990s. However, the first large-scale randomised clinical trial to track hormone therapy in healthy postmenopausal women – the Women's Health Initiative (WHI) – was stopped earlier than planned, as researchers found that the health risks of the trial exceeded the health benefits; they were found to be at increased risk of developing breast cancer. The publication of this result in 2002 in the *British Medical Journal* (BMJ)[1] caused panic among many women on HRT and doctors were advised to stop prescribing it. However, it later emerged that the findings of the WHI study were unreliable, as a majority of the study participants were more than a decade beyond the menopause transition, that is, they were already at a higher risk for breast cancer. The risk of breast cancer from HRT is now considered very small with the benefits outweighing the risks. However, HRT continues to be quite polarising with regard to a 'medicalised' vs 'natural' standpoint.

At present, HRT is the most widely used medical treatment for menopausal symptoms, with around 15% of women aged 45 to 64 in England currently prescribed HRT.[2] Overall, it is thought to be a safe and effective treatment for most women. However, there are some for whom HRT is unsuitable due to increased risks associated with certain types of cancer, such as breast and endometrial cancer, or other medical complications.

If you are considering taking HRT, you should have a good discussion with your GP and talk through the options, so they can advise on the balance of risks against benefits of taking it, based on your medical history.

Non-hormonal medical treatments

Some women cannot take HRT. And there are others who don't want to for various reasons, opting for non-hormonal medicine or alternative therapies instead. Even a brief search online brings up a wide range of non-hormonal and alternative treatments suggested for relief from menopausal symptoms. But, of course, it is important that the knowledge we gain is based on sound, evidence-based information, in order to make informed choices about how to manage our symptoms. There is evidence for non-hormonal medical treatments, which are effective in treating vasomotor symptoms,[3] and there are new medicines being developed too.[4] I found a review paper by two highly respected London-based consultant gynaecologists, Veronica Djpardy and Nick Panay,[3] very informative in this respect. Professor Panay is currently the president of the International Menopause Society and previously the chair of the British Menopause Society.

Djpardy and Panay looked into the effectiveness of alternative and non-hormonal treatments though they have focused only on vasomotor symptoms (hot flushes and night sweats) and vaginal atrophy (dryness).[3] They discuss non-hormonal medical treatments such as: antidepressants called selective serotonin-reuptake inhibitors (SSRIs) and serotonin and norepinephrine reuptake inhibitors (SNRIs); Clonidine; Gabapentin; and Pregabalin. With all medications, there are side effects to take into consideration, especially if they have the potential to interact with other medication. Also, some side effects might make other menopausal symptoms worse, such as those causing difficulty sleeping, putting on weight, or sexual dysfunction. So again, you need to discuss with your doctor to weigh up the benefits against the risks.

Cognitive behavioural therapy (CBT)

This is a psychological therapy that enables us to become more aware of our thoughts, emotions, physical reactions and behaviours, and understand how they are all linked. That is, the way we interpret situations and think about things has an impact on how we behave and how we feel about that situation. CBT helps us to see where our patterns of thinking and reacting might not be helpful and helps us develop practical ways to manage difficult situations by learning skills and techniques for coping.

I will be discussing the implementation of CBT principles and strategies throughout this book. CBT has been shown to be effective in improving the emotional and physical symptoms of menopause, including stress, anxiety, low mood, sleep problems, hot flushes and night sweats, mainly by changing your cognitive appraisal of the experienced symptoms. A number of randomised controlled trials, led by Professor Myra Hunter, Emeritus Professor of Clinical Health Psychology at King's College London, have demonstrated that CBT (delivered either as self-help or group therapy) reduces the impact of problematic hot flushes and night sweats by an average of 50%. In addition, the CBT intervention also improved their rating with regard to mood and memory problems, and significantly improved the women's quality of life.[5,6] CBT is recommended as an effective non-hormonal treatment for vasomotor symptoms by The North American Menopause Society,[7] the British Menopause Society[8] and the in the NICE guidelines (see below).

Complementary and alternative remedies, practices and therapies

Many of us prefer to try out more natural approaches first and think that if those work, we will stick with them, but if symptoms persist, we might consider HRT or other medication if permitted by our medical history or after weighing up the benefits over the risks. Reviews of studies in the USA and the UK have found that around half of menopausal women turn to complementary and alternative approaches.[2,9] These are also discussed in Djpardy and Panay's review paper.

Natural approaches may refer to self-management or lifestyle in terms of diet and exercise, dietary supplements, herbal remedies, homeopathic remedies, Ayuverdic medicine, traditional Chinese medicine and other complementary approaches such as mindfulness and yoga.

Mindfulness – This is a technique which involves being still and fully immersed in the present moment while accepting without judgement what you are thinking. Recent research from the Mayo Clinic in Minnesota has shown that menopausal women who practised mindfulness suffered less with anxiety, irritability and depression.[10] I will discuss mindfulness further in Chapter 6.

Yoga The roots of yoga are in Indian philosophy as a spiritual practice. These days, it is widely practiced in the Western world for its physical postures, breathing techniques and meditation. As there are many different types of yoga practice, it can be difficult to compare across research studies to evaluate the health benefits of yoga. However, there is scientific evidence to suggest that the practice of yoga leads to benefits in numerous aspects of physical health and mental wellbeing, including managing stress; maintaining mental/emotional health; improvements in strength, balance and flexibility; and promoting better quality of sleep.[11,12] A systematic review of 13 studies, including 1306 participants, concluded that yoga seems to be at least as effective as other types of exercise in relieving menopause symptoms. Yoga practice was found to reduce physical symptoms such as hot flushes as well as psychological symptoms such as anxiety or depression.[13] It may be that, like meditation and relaxation exercises, it helps lower the cortisol level in the body, making women less stressed, and so less sensitive to hot flushes. I have been practicing yoga on and off for years because I feel good physically and mentally for doing it. As it has been shown to be effective and safe for reducing menopausal symptoms by some research, I would say if you enjoy it, stick with it, even if only for the overall health benefits.

Over-the-counter products – There seem to be a fast-growing market of products aimed at menopausal women. Among them is a wide array of herbal remedies suggested to be used in combination with or as an alternative to conventional medicine. We tend to assume they are harmless because they come from natural sources, but this may not necessarily be the case. Some herbs can react in your body to cause unwanted effects and may potentially cause risk by interacting with other medications. Also, as there are no recognised international criteria for testing them – like those that exist for conventional medicine – it can be hard to conclude that they are effective and safe. There is a European Union (EU) Directive for the registration of traditional herbal medicinal products and approved products are marked with the THR (Traditional Herbal Remedy) certification mark/logo on the packaging.

Regarding the above-mentioned alternative and complimentary approaches, as so many women do use them and report relief from symptoms as a result of using them, further research is warranted. On the whole, we need more scientific evidence for their safety and effectiveness in managing menopausal symptoms. As Djapady and Panay state, although some complementary remedies are shown to have insufficient scientific evidence to back them up, it does not mean they do not actually work; it just means they have not been proven to work with large enough samples. We need more well-designed studies with large numbers of participants to provide the scientific backing to give us the confidence to use them. My personal view is that if I hear lots of women say something helped them, I will check that they are not harmful and look for evidence of their efficacy, check they don't interact with my existing medication, look for the best source of the product and give it a go for about three months, as long as it doesn't cost an arm and a leg. But, of course, you should consult with your doctor before trying any complementary treatment.

NICE guidelines for the treatment of menopause

In England, there is an independent organisation called the National Institute for Health and Care Excellence (NICE), which was set up by the government in 1999. NICE sets out guidelines based on evidence-based research and consultation with experts in relevant fields, to provide recommendations for treatment approaches and care services for people with a specific condition or need. Most clinicians abide by these guidelines as much as possible. The NICE guideline for menopause were published in November 2015,[14] and last updated in December 2019. A newly updated guideline is in development and expected to be published at the end of 2024.

Health professionals are advised to adopt an individualised approach in the diagnosis and management of perimenopause and menopause. They are advised to diagnose according to the age of the woman and taking into account other conditions or needs. Although, blood tests for diagnosis is not recommended for women over 45, it is suggested that for women aged 40 to 45 years with menopausal symptoms or those under 40 years in whom menopause is suspected, diagnosis may be confirmed by two blood tests for FSH level taken four to six weeks apart.

HRT is recommended for the medical management of menopausal symptoms. CBT has been proven to be effective in reducing the frequency and severity of hot flushes and night sweats, and is recommended to be considered alongside or as an alternative to HRT. Both HRT and CBT are advised to be considered for low mood related to menopause and CBT for anxiety.

Women should be advised about all treatment options so they can select that which may work best for them, weighing up the risks and benefits with the help of their doctor. NICE says the evidence on HRT has become clearer since the last guidance in 2015. And if they opt for HRT, it is advised to use the lowest effective dose. Women started on treatment should be reviewed regularly and treatment adapted according to the response to the treatment or change in symptoms.

As for complementary therapies, NICE recommends that women should be informed that the quality, purity and constituents of products may be unknown.

Full details of the recommendations can be found by searching 'NICE guidelines on menopause' online. If you are living in England, and generally in the UK, this information should help you be informed about the treatment you can expect and request from your GP.

My experience with supplements

I will share here my 'experiment' with supplements as anecdotal evidence to demonstrate an example of the lived experience – the process of weighing up my options and making decisions.

It can be quite overwhelming when you go shopping for supplements, as I found one afternoon when I went to see what was on offer, in the midst of a period of bad hot flushes and joint pain. I had done some research beforehand, but still was not sure what I 'needed' when faced by a huge display of products, all promising to alleviate/relieve my symptoms of menopause. After doing all my checks, I made a choice with the attitude of 'it's worth a try'. By the time I finished my first pack (26 days), I believed I had had fewer hot flushes and although I was still getting a bit hot in bed, I had not been so hot to be sweating into my clothes. I decided to continue onto another pack to be sure they were effective. Into my sixth week of being on the supplements, I noticed that I hadn't had a single hot-flush during the day for a few weeks. I was still sticking my feet out of the covers in bed when a little over-heated – though that was my habit before perimenopause – but was not sweating at all.

Of course, it could just be a coincidence that the hot flushes and night sweats stopped at this time and not scientific evidence that the supplements worked. I did consider possible confounding variables (other things that might have played a part), but I had not started my diet and exercise routine at this stage nor was I using anything else. I couldn't think of any other changes I had made which might have accounted for the reduction in hot flushes and night sweats. So, I decided to do a little experiment where I would come off them after my third pack (after almost three months) to see if my symptoms returned. Just over two weeks later, I found myself asking, 'Is it me or is it hot in here?' again and noticed the hot flushes and night sweats were creeping back. Having got used to not having them, I was now finding them more intolerable and dreading them returning in full force. As nothing else had changed, I assumed the effect of the supplements must have worn off.

Now I decided I had two options – I could just go back on the supplements, or I thought, rather than take the supplements, why not try and incorporate the ingredients they contained in the natural form in my diet. But, of course, I quickly realised that the supplements have the ingredients in concentrated doses, and I'd have to drink bucket-loads of herbal tea and eat truck-loads of the other ingredients to get the amounts I needed. So, I opted to go back on the supplements. Maybe there is a placebo effect – my mind telling me they worked – but on an individual level, I believe there is actually nothing wrong with this. If it works for me, it works for me. Maybe the supplements are helping, maybe the hot flushes and night sweats went away naturally with the fluctuations in my hormones, maybe they've just gone for a while and will be back. Whatever the reason, I was happy to pay the cost of the supplements for the relief I felt for now. But it also doesn't mean that I shouldn't make the effort to incorporate the helpful nutrients into my diet for extra support. This has been my experience so far, but if you are considering taking supplements, you may want to consult with your doctor depending on your personal medical history.

Key points

Do your research, from reliable sources, before deciding which treatment approaches to try.

Always get medical advice in the context of your personal medical history

Today I am grateful for:

My professional training in scrutinising research studies

My CBT and other self-management skills

The privilege of choice - for different treatment options

Your turn:

List your **key learning points** from this chapter

List two or three things (big or small) you are **grateful for** right now

4 Taking a Holistic Approach

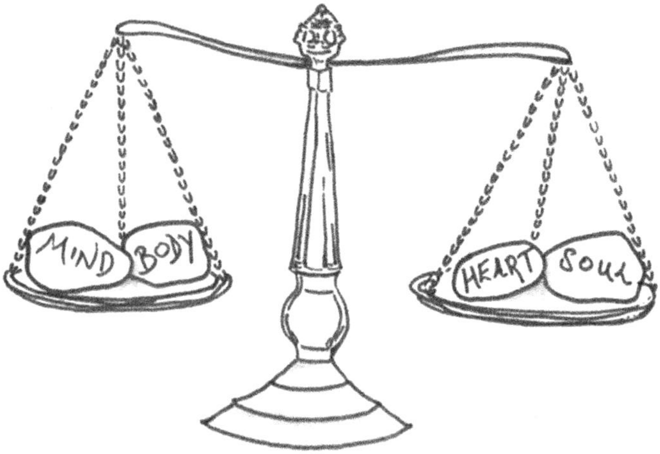

Before we go on to the practical application of psychological approaches for managing our menopausal symptoms, let's look at how we might understand this process of transition and put it into some sort of perspective.

As we have seen from the descriptions so far, there is a wide range of symptoms that the menopausal process can throw at us. And we will see that it can impact on our whole lives in a variety of ways – mentally, physically, at work and in our relationships. Also, we know that there is not a uniform course that we all take on this path, that is, our experiences of the menopause can vary greatly. So, it follows that when we want to make sense of what's happening to us and consider how we might manage the symptoms, we need to take a multidimensional perspective. We need to be aware of the biological processes at play and the medical approaches to understanding and managing symptoms; we need to consider the psychological processes and models for coping; and we also need to be aware of the impact of social influences. This is usually described as a biopsychosocial approach.

The biopsychosocial model was introduced to the world of medical practice and training of health professionals by George L. Engel in 1977,[1] who proposed that doctors should simultaneously take into account the biological, psychological and social aspects of illness. He believed that this approach helped the medical profession to better understand the patient's subjective experience of their illness and led to more accurate diagnosis, more humane care and improved health outcomes. This idea was further developed to value the patient–clinician relationship and empower the patient in clinical decision-making in their treatment. Menopause is not a disease or illness, but there is no denying that it does cause women to go through a number of changes and experience symptoms which need to be effectively managed. So, taking a biopsychosocial perspective to consider all aspects of the menopausal transition that impact on us, can help us find effective coping strategies. This approach encourages empowerment and joint decision-making with our healthcare providers regarding our treatment.

My biopsychosocial-spiritual model

With regard to menopause, I would like to take the biopsychosocial model a step further and propose a more holistic approach. In addition to simultaneously taking into account the biological, psychological and social aspects of the menopause experience, I propose that we add spirituality into the mix. I believe, and this is supported by research, that the additional element of spirituality can be very beneficial to coping, where it is a meaningful part of a woman's life.

So, what is spirituality? 'Spirituality' can be a difficult concept to describe, as it can mean different things to different people. Broadly speaking, it is the belief in something beyond the self and what we experience on a physical and sensory level, exploring feelings of interconnectedness and seeking meaning and purpose in life. For some people, their spirituality is tied in with a belief in God and active participation in organised religion. For others, it involves non-religious and non-theistic concepts like the power of positive thinking, practices such as yoga, meditation or spending time in nature.

Psychologists often like to represent their ideas with diagrams, which we call models. In Figure 4.1 below, I have drawn a simple diagram to show how I make sense of the menopause from a holistic perspective. The idea is that it encompasses the whole experience, that is, all the different elements that make up my menopause experience. I have called it a biopsychosocial-spiritual model for understanding the process of menopause and how we might tackle the management of our symptoms. These concepts will explain my approach to managing the menopausal transition. I hope you can relate to this model as it is. However, if you feel you have no inclination towards spirituality at all, you can leave that part out and see the 'meno and me' part of the model as being simply about your self-identity and personal values.

I have always considered myself to be a spiritual person, both in the general interpretation of the concept as well as in a more religious sense. Though my practice of my religion has fluctuated over the years, as is common, my personal values are very much based on it. If this was not a book about my own lived experience and I was writing about coping strategies only from the professional stance of a clinical psychologist, I would likely not mention my faith and its influence on my coping

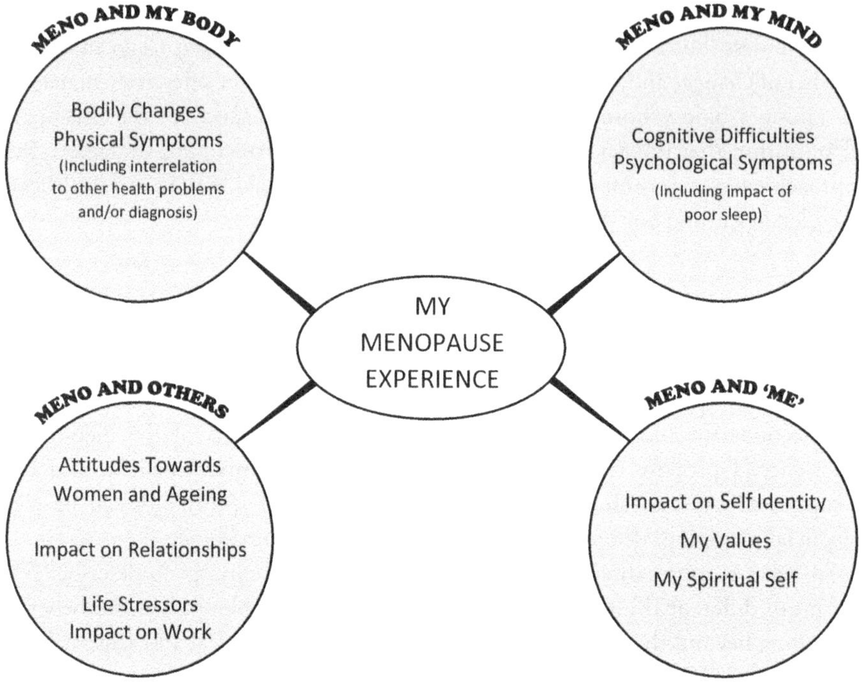

FIGURE 4.1 Biopsychosocial-Spiritual Model of the Menopause Experience

with the menopause. But it *is* about me and my personal experiences, so I believe it would not be authentic if I omitted the influence of my faith and spiritual sensibilities where they are relevant to my coping.

During my training as a clinical psychologist in the late 1990s, I do not recall much, if any, mention of spirituality, and even now, spirituality features very little, if at all, in most training courses. This might suggest that it is not considered an important factor in people's understanding and resolving of their personal problems. However, there is plenty of research indicating otherwise. It has been shown that those who are religious or spiritual and use their spirituality to cope with challenges in life experience many positive outcomes in their health and wellbeing.[2]

Spirituality has also been linked to increased compassion, psychological wellbeing and life satisfaction.[3] Religious and spiritual interventions have been correlated with better physical and mental health, including increased immunity, lower blood pressure and an overall lower rate of mortality.[4] The attitudes and practices of spirituality and faith can be a valuable resource of strength and hope. They can help us to reduce the emotional distress caused by adverse life events, such as loss or change, by giving meaning to suffering, and so making it more bearable. They can help us regulate stress and allow for more acceptance when things are out of our personal control. When we belong to an organised religious group, we may benefit from the sense of community that it offers and the social support, especially at difficult times like during a bereavement.

I think we generally tend to think of the Eastern world as more spiritual (and disparagingly, less scientific) and the Western world less spiritual and more scientific. Coming from an Eastern background but growing up in a Western society, I am in the advantageous position, where I am able to see things from both perspectives and take the best from each. And having straddled both worlds has enabled me to be more comfortable to take a holistic approach to treatments in my personal life. It also opens up the opportunity for my clients to bring their ethnic and cultural values, spirituality and faith into the work we are doing together, if and when they want to. I have also done some training in Islamic approaches to psychology and psychotherapy and was amazed to discover that many of the ideas I learnt during my training in Western psychology in the UK, already existed many years ago in the Islamic world.[5] I think the main difference between Western psychology and Islamic psychology is that where the former focuses on the mind, the latter additionally also incorporates the heart and soul into its psychological models – a more holistic approach.

So, along with the biological, psychological and social elements that make up my menopausal experience, I will, on occasion, mention how my spiritual outlook has helped with the menopausal transition, in case it helps others, to see things from such a perspective. However, although my personal practices might have an underlying faith element to them, if you prefer, you can use the strategies in this book without them having any connection to spirituality or faith.

There are many health and wellbeing practices – for example, yoga – which have now become everyday practices but are often separated from their original source of spirituality. While in the Western world, psychological theories have tended to 'stand-alone' or 'apart' from spirituality or faith, some current psychological approaches actually originate from such backgrounds, such as mindfulness from Buddhism and meditation which is a part of life in many Eastern religions. It is respectful to give due credit to the source of such knowledge and practice though I think most of us believe it is acceptable to utilise them to our benefit without the spiritual or faith link.

Introduction to psychological approaches for self-management

Psychological theories are developed from hypotheses about human behaviour which are tested with research, seeking evidence to validate them where appropriate. They describe how humans behave under certain conditions and make predictions about how they might behave in the future under particular circumstances. Psychological models for ways to address different conditions are usually drawn from a range of such theories from different schools of thought, such as behavioural, cognitive, psychodynamic and humanistic theories of psychology.

Approaches for managing and treating symptoms rely on the idea that: (i) people can be supported in becoming aware of and reporting on their health complaints and (ii) people can set goals and adjust them according to skills learnt, reviewing progress and reflections on the experience. This kind of self-awareness and self-regulation is needed for good self-care management and collaboration with health professionals in managing our care. As menopause is not a mental health condition, it does not require a treatment model as such. However, we can draw on various theoretical ideas to plan how we might cope with all that it throws at us in terms of psychological symptoms and the secondary effects of the physical symptoms.

Cognitive behaviour therapy (CBT)

The practice of cognitive behaviour therapy (CBT) – or cognitive therapy as it started out as a form of psychotherapy – was developed in the 1960s by Aaron T. Beck. Up until then, behaviour therapy helped patients make sense of their difficulties by observing their behavioural responses to stimuli. Beck realised that it was not sufficient to simply observe a patient's response to stimuli, but it was necessary to ask what happens in the step in between – what were the patient's thoughts (cognitions)? Beck observed that his patients with depression often described thoughts that seemed to 'lack validity' and seemed to be 'distorted'. He believed that working with these 'cognitive distortions' in their thinking was the key to helping them understand themselves and make sense of things. Having demonstrated the efficacy of cognitive therapy, he set out his ideas as a treatment protocol in his book, 'Cognitive Therapy for Depression'.[6]

Over the years, CBT has become the most extensively researched of all psychotherapies, and so it is now the main evidence-based treatment approach for a wide range of psychological problems, such as anxiety, depression, substance abuse, eating disorders and anger management. It also has been found to be effective in helping people cope with the impact of an array of physical health conditions, such as chronic fatigue syndrome, fibromyalgia, irritable bowel syndrome, insomnia, migraines and other chronic pain conditions.

The focus of CBT is on the link between our cognitions (this refers to the whole range of internal mental processes – thoughts, images, memories, urges and impulses), emotions and behaviours. It is based on the idea that in a given situation, the interpretations we make about the situation has more of an influence on how we react to it – in terms of our feelings, behaviour and physical responses – than the situation itself; also, that our interpretations may be unrealistic, inaccurate or unhelpful. Such interpretations are called 'negative automatic thoughts', and they are thought to be driven by unhelpful underlying rules or assumptions we have for living our life and deeper beliefs that we hold about ourselves, about others and the world in general. The essence of CBT is to help us to recognise, challenge and change the unhelpful patterns of thoughts and behaviours that can make us feel anxious, depressed or distressed. The aim is to enable us to have a more realistic outlook, better manage our emotions and change our behaviours, and so deal more effectively with the stresses and problems in our lives.

With regard to coping during the menopausal transition, there is a good evidence-base for the use of CBT to manage symptoms, as discussed in Chapter 3. I will show you a range of CBT-based strategies you can use. You will be able to see how your thoughts and reactions to your menopausal symptoms might be affecting the way you end up feeling about yourself, and how making sometimes fairly small changes could have a positive impact not only on how you manage your symptoms, but also your overall sense of wellbeing.

Acceptance and commitment therapy (ACT)

The original behavioural and cognitive approaches to psychotherapy have expanded so that there are now numerous other approaches which come under the umbrella of cognitive-behavioural therapies and are called third-wave behavioural approaches. They are more focused on looking at the context and processes of our thoughts and actions by learning to notice and accept them before making attempts at any change that we may feel is needed, where change is possible. Third wave therapies incorporate components such as: mindfulness; acceptance; self-awareness; self-compassion; spirituality; and actions driven by personal values.

Acceptance and commitment therapy (ACT – articulated as the word 'act') is one of the more prominent third-wave therapies. It was developed in the 1980s by Professor Steven C. Hayes[7] and has been extensively written about and developed by Dr. Russ Harris.[8] There are three core functional components to ACT, specifically:

1. accepting what we have and cannot change
2. choosing to live life according to our values
3. taking action to live a meaningful life in line with our values

As a spiritual person of faith, I think ACT as a psychological therapy approach probably comes closest to allowing me to incorporate my beliefs and values system with psychological tools, and that's perhaps why I personally feel comfortable using this approach.

The key aim of ACT is to develop and expand what Hayes calls 'psychological flexibility'. This means learning to become aware of our thoughts and feelings, stepping back from them and observing them and adapting our behaviours to be in line with our values. Sometimes our difficulties can arise from avoiding, denying and struggling with our inner feelings. ACT teaches us to accept that these deeper emotional responses are appropriate to certain situations and that acknowledging and accepting them does not mean we can't move forward with our life. So, the name 'acceptance and commitment' therapy is based on the idea that we can accept our difficulties and commit to taking the necessary actions to change things, regardless of what is going on in our life or how we feel about it. We do this by engaging in mindfulness and using experiential exercises and metaphors. An essential feature in the ACT approach is to identify our personal values and set our goals to align with our values, with the aim of achieving a meaningful life.

As you will see in the upcoming chapters on coping strategies, I have used this approach to help me put my menopause experience into perspective, not struggle with it so much and feel more able to manage the symptoms. I will show you the tools for putting the ACT process in operation for your own experience.

My integrative approach to therapy and life

As a clinical psychologist, I tend to take an integrative approach in my work with clients. This means drawing from a number of theoretical approaches I have been trained in and tailoring the methods used to the individual needs of the client. I develop and share my hypotheses about what might be going on for the client and collaborate with them on how to implement changes using appropriate therapeutic techniques that are scientifically proven to be effective for the problems we have identified. In this way, I am not restricted to, nor suggesting that only one approach can work for every situation. I think this is the approach we all tend to take in managing our lives.

As with any task at hand, the tools we use will depend on the problem we are trying to solve and what we believe will do the best job. For menopausal symptoms, cognitive behavioural therapy (CBT) has so far been shown to be the most effective and efficient approach, and it is also my area of specialism. So, that is where many of the tools and strategies that I will be sharing with you will have been derived from. I think of CBT as a common sense, structured and systematic approach. Although the focus is on problem solving in the here and now, I think, in most cases, it also helps to take a deeper look at how the problem developed over time and gain an understanding of how to not let the unhelpful aspects of the past continue to dictate the future. Menopause can be a time when we start to re-evaluate our lives, so we may need to give space to understanding how things developed over time.

ACT is a more values-based approach, which has an evidence base in relation to physical health and can be helpful when we are facing situations, which we have little control over. And for some, in addition to these approaches, it helps to explore things in the context of their spiritual and/or faith values and framework, of course, only where this is relevant and desired by the client. In this way, I believe I am taking a holistic approach to helping my clients. And of course, the same applies to myself for dealing with the everyday challenges in life, as well as for the management of my menopausal symptoms.

Mind-mapping – a tool for keeping tabs on symptoms and coping strategies

The biopsychosocial-spiritual model in Figure 4.2 is like an overall representation of my menopause experience. To consider coping strategies, the next step would be to look at each area in more detail. One of the most difficult things about the menopausal experience is that there can be so much going on at once, making it all feel quite overwhelming. Whenever I have a lot going on in my head and am trying to process it all, or when I have a lot of tasks or plans in different aspects of my life, which is often, I turn to mind-mapping. The concept of communicating complex categories using a tree-like map is thought to date back to the Greek philosopher, Porphyry, around 330A.D.[9] Tony Buzan described the concept of mind-mapping as we use it today.[10] I got into mind-mapping after taking my children to a workshop on it at the Science Museum, and since then, I've always got a mind map on the go, not only for personal projects but also for developing formulations and treatment plans for my client work.[11] They work for me because I'm quite a visual thinker, and I like to see things laid out on one page.

I have found the mind map particularly useful for setting out all my menopausal symptoms in one place. It's not just the symptoms being so varied and unpredictable that makes the whole experience difficult, but also that it's hard to keep up with how to manage them. As the symptoms keep shifting, trying to manage them can

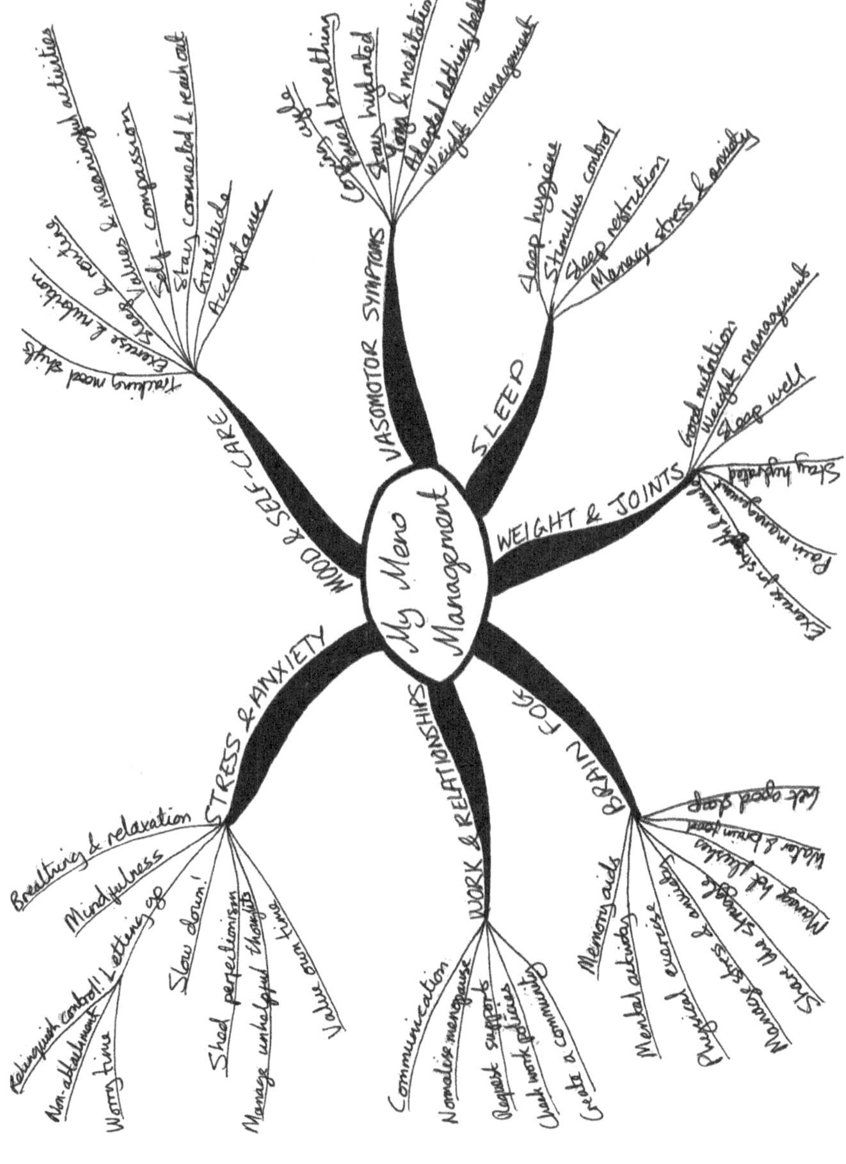

FIGURE 4.2 Mind Map of the Menopause Experience and Coping Solutions

feel like shooting at a moving target. For example, I might have just got to grips with keeping the hot flushes at bay, when the joint pains return, and I feel I am back to square one, needing to remember how to manage that. Add the impact of brain fog and anxiety into the mix, and you can see how frustrating and overwhelming it can feel. By using the mind map, when I had worked out helpful strategies for managing a symptom, I can put that down. Then, when the symptom is not bothering me for a while, I can forget about it, confident that if it comes back, I can check what I had found effective before and re-apply that, rather than having to start problem-solving from scratch.

So, this is the first tool I am sharing with you. Figure 4.2 shows a mind map of my symptoms and coping solutions. You can use or adapt this one, or better still draw up your own to reflect your symptoms and solutions as you progress through your menopausal journey. You might like to see it as a tool for organising your thoughts and putting things into perspective. Just include the bits that are relevant for you and leave out those that are not. I still like to do my mind maps on paper, as I feel more 'connected' to them that way, but if you prefer to do it digitally, there are mobile apps available.

Key points

Menopause is experienced by the whole 'you' - so take a holistic approach to living through it

CBT and ACT are effective psychological approaches

Mind maps are fun to draw and a helpful way to keep tabs on symptoms and solutions

Today I am grateful for:

My spirituality and faith-based grounding for life

My training and experience in a range of therapeutic approaches

Having access to a range of helpful tools to manage my symptoms

Your turn:

List your **key learning points** from this chapter

List two or three things (big or small) you are **grateful for** right now

Part II

Symptoms and Coping Strategies

5 Menopause and Mental Health

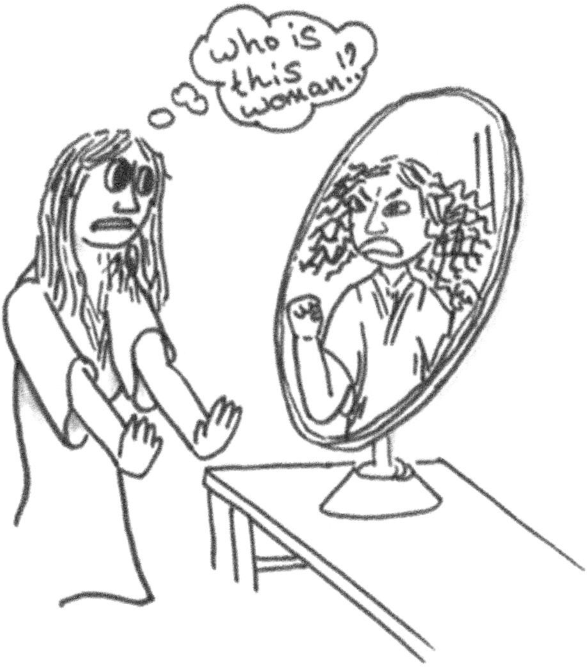

Although the menopausal transition is a biological process that leads to bodily changes and physical symptoms, for many of us, the psychological symptoms and emotional turmoil can be just as challenging and play havoc with our lives. Often, when we are not aware that we are perimenopausal and/or don't know that psychological symptoms are a part of the process, we become very confused about what is going on with us. We may feel like we are 'going crazy' when we have sudden emotional outbursts or dramatic mood shifts or not understand why we've become so anxious about everything lately. Menopause can be a really challenging time for our mental health, with one recent large survey finding 69% of women experience difficulties with anxiety and depression due to menopause.[1]

Differentiating between stress, anxiety and worry

The words stress and anxiety often get used interchangeably, and the same goes for anxiety and worry. But there are differences between them. Stress is a physiological response typically caused by an external trigger, a stressor – for example, an upcoming work deadline or awaiting the results of an important medical test. The stress response is our body's natural way of reacting to a threat. The body under stress fires up the limbic system and releases the hormones adrenaline and cortisol, which help activate the brain and body to deal with the threat. Signs of stress in the body include a rapid heart rate, clammy palms and shallow breath. When the threat/difficult situation is over, our body relaxes. This is called acute stress, and the body's reaction actually serves a positive function in keeping us safe. While we might be able to manage short bursts of stress and might even feel good when the adrenaline and cortisol flood our body and help us overcome a difficult situation or achieve something significant, if it goes on for prolonged periods, we are at risk of suffering from chronic stress problems. When chronically stressed, the body stays in this fight-or-flight mode continuously (usually because the difficult situation has not resolved, such as ongoing problems at work or financial strains) and this can lead to psychological problems, such as irritability, anger, fatigue, and difficulty sleeping, as well as physical health problems, such as muscle pain, digestive issues, a weakening of the immune system or an increased risk of heart disease.

Anxiety is also a natural response to a threat, but this time, there is no actual threat – it is a perceived threat. Think of a scenario where you arrive at an event and feel that you don't fit in. You may think someone looked at you as if they didn't like you or looked like they disapproved of what you are wearing. You will start to have all the physiology of a stress response because you're telling yourself that you are being judged, which might *feel* like a threat. You might feel hot, think you are visibly going red and feel the urge to get away as your body is in a state of fight or flight – but there is no real threat here, you don't know that they are judging you and you don't need to escape to save yourself.

Worry is what is going on in our mind when we are anxious. Worries tend to be repetitive, obsessive thoughts that occur when we are uncertain about outcomes or predict something might go wrong. These are 'What if?' kind of thoughts. So, anxiety has a cognitive element (worry) and a physiological element (stress response), hence, we experience anxiety in both our mind and body.

Despite these differences, mild-to-moderate stress and anxiety respond well to similar coping strategies. So, I will use the words interchangeably when referring to management tools for them.

How anxiety presents in menopause

Menopausal anxiety – The prevalence rates of anxiety during the menopausal transition has been reported to be anything from 9 to 58% depending on the size of the sample studies, the inclusion criteria used and the anxiety rating scale used.[2] Although women may have experienced anxiety before they started their menopausal transition, it has been found that even among women who did not have anxiety before, there was a greater likelihood of reporting anxiety now compared to when they were premenopausal. And that's even when other potential anxiety-inducing factors, like upsetting or stressful life events, have been accounted for.[3]

Menopause-related anxiety is different from other types of anxiety in that it ebbs and flows with fluctuations in hormones, as I'll explain below. It can also occur in response to menopausal symptoms. The unpredictability of symptoms, such as hot flushes for example, can make you anxious about when they will occur and how you will cope. For some women, the sudden onset of hot flushes in the presence of others can cause embarrassment, which can also lead to a sense of panic, maybe even panic attacks. When these occur unexpectedly or suddenly and are experienced frequently, you may develop panic disorder, the main feature of which is being anxious about having a panic attack. This is reported by many women during menopause. Although there may be a range of factors that can lead to a panic attack, being more susceptible to anxiety at this stage, may be considered a likely contributor.

Not knowing when symptoms will strike and when they might be more severe than usual can also make you anxious about making commitments. For example, when you don't know when your heavy periods will appear and exactly how heavy they'll be or when your hot flushes might be at their worst. Sometimes you may have no choice about agreeing to do things into the future and can be anxious for some time beforehand. For example, I often have to commit months in advance to giving lectures at the university. If my symptoms are bad in the run up to the lecture, I can get anxious about how I'll manage on the day.

Palpitations – A recent study has reported that half of us are likely to experience a 'sustained low probability' of palpitations during the menopausal transition, with the highest likelihood being during perimenopause and early postmenopause. And these palpitations were not associated with subclinical cardiovascular disease.[4] Although menopausal palpitations are physiological, occurring when oestrogen drops and sometimes during a hot flush, they have psychological consequences in that they often lead to feelings of dread, panic, anxiety or fear of heart attacks. My husband once called emergency services for me at 2 a.m., thinking I was having a heart attack when I was actually experiencing palpitations. The paramedics insisted on taking me to hospital for further tests (my first time in an ambulance, aged 48), and after spending the night at the accident and emergencies department, I was glad they found nothing wrong with my heart. However, they also gave me no other possible explanation for my symptoms.

Fear of embarrassment or social judgement – Worrying about what others will think can cause you to have anticipatory anxiety. This is being anxious about what you *think* might happen and how you *might* react even before anything actually happens. You can get anxious that a hot flush may suddenly show up when you are around others or an episode of brain fog might make you fumble around for words or going completely blank when communicating with others and worrying that you won't cope in the situation or will leave a bad impression. Anticipatory anxiety puts you on edge and holds you back even before you encounter the situation.

Mood-related symptoms

Mood swings – Many of us may already be familiar with our mood being affected by our menstrual cycles, such as feeling tearful, irritable, anxious or low in mood. But during the menopause, mood changes may feel even worse. We may experience a sudden shift in mood and find ourselves feeling tearful, sad or angry, for no apparent reason and be unable to identify any immediate triggers. These sudden outbursts of emotion can be confusing and take an emotional toll on us, as well as impacting those close to us. For those who have a history of bipolar disorder, studies have demonstrated an increased likelihood of mood fluctuations during the late menopause transition and early postmenopause stage.[5]

Tearfulness, irritability and anger – With so much going on in our bodies – hot flushes, aches and pains, and lack of sleep – it is not surprising that we can also feel tearful, low in mood, cranky and maybe even prone to bursts of anger.

Low mood or depression – Several large prospective cohort studies (that is, research which follows a group of people over time) have found that we are at an increased risk of experiencing low mood when going through menopause. Data across numerous studies found that depressive symptoms are reported by 45 to 68% of perimenopausal women, compared to 28 to 31% of women who have not started on their menopausal journey.[6] It has also been shown that we are at three times the risk for developing clinical depression when we are in perimenopause, compared to when we are premenopausal.[7] Most women who experience clinical depression during perimenopause have experienced a prior episode of depression. So, one or more previous episodes of depression increases the risk of future episodes during perimenopause.[8]

Other risk factors for perimenopausal depression include a previous history of severe premenstrual syndrome (PMS) – the symptoms women can experience prior to their period; premenstrual dysphoric disorder (PMDD) – an extreme form of PMS with severe emotional and physical symptoms; postnatal depression – which some women experience in the first year after giving birth;[9] as well as prior anxiety disorder, life stresses and other health conditions.[8]

Menopausal symptoms can complicate, co-occur, and overlap with the presentation of primary clinical (or 'typical') depression. Menopause-related depression is different from premenopausal clinical depression in that it is affected by fluctuations in our hormones. But it can be difficult to distinguish between symptoms caused by typical depression and those caused by underlying hormonal changes. Some suggestions put forward to help in differentiating between them include:[10]

- In perimenopausal depression, women often describe the symptoms as coming and going from day to day, and symptoms may be worse in the morning and before periods.
- In typical depression, there is not so much fluctuation in symptoms although there may be an improvement in mood in the evenings.
- In perimenopausal depression, there will be the presence of other menopausal symptoms and not the reduced appetite and weight loss that might be present in typical depression.
- Women themselves might describe their perimenopausal depression as being similar to PMS, or if they have had premenopausal clinical depression, they might describe their symptoms as feeling different this time.

For diagnostic purposes, doctors will need to investigate the individual woman's mental health history, make an assessment of any co-occurring psychiatric and menopausal symptoms (e.g., enquire about oestrogen and testosterone deficiency symptoms), take into account psychosocial factors common in midlife (for example, life stressors such as caring for ageing parents), and can also use validated screening instruments such as the MENO-D[11] and the Green Climacteric Scale.[12] Until they clarify what the underlying cause of the presenting depression symptoms is, it can be difficult for a doctor to decide on the treatment approach to take. For typical depression the main treatment approaches are antidepressants and/or psychological therapy (CBT). For perimenopausal depression, depending on whether they think there is a co-occurrence with typical depression, they may offer HRT, antidepressants, psychological therapy, or a combination of these.[13]

Suicidalilty – There has been increasing concern about data from around the world showing that women are at highest risk for suicide during midlife.[10,14,15] In the UK, women aged 45–54 years have the highest suicide rate.[16] A survey of 2,000 women in the UK found that 1 in 10 reported experiencing suicidal thoughts which they attributed to perimenopause,[17] indicating that for some women, their symptoms may be so severe and debilitating that they will contemplate ending their life. Though there is limited research and no clear indication of a causal link between menopause and suicidality, it has been suggested that there may be some association with biological changes during menopause.[10]

There is further information on where to seek help for mental health problems in the Further Support and Resources section at the back.

What causes menopausal anxiety and mood problems?

Fluctuating hormone levels – Changes in the levels of oestrogen, progesterone and testosterone in our body has an impact on our brain and mood. Oestrogen stimulates the production of a mood-boosting chemical called serotonin, which regulates our state of mind and anxiety levels. It also plays a role in the production of endorphins, a chemical which soothes our body and enables us to feel good. So, a decline in the oestrogen level in the body can have a significant impact on how we feel. Progesterone has a mildly sedative effect on our brain and body and so it relaxes us. A drop in progesterone levels causes our body to release the stress hormones cortisol and adrenaline, which make us feel anxious and irritable. It is when this process happens quickly that extreme emotions or sudden outbursts get triggered. The role of testosterone in our brain is to improve mood, energy and motivation, so a drop in this can lead to us feeling flat or deflated. Researchers have also found that drops in oestrogen levels in perimenopausal women can make us prone to increase in levels of a brain protein called monoamine oxidase A, which is also linked to depression.[18]

Secondary effects of physical symptoms The numerous physical symptoms of hot flushes, night sweats, muscles aches, joint pains, as well as the lack of sleep that these and other issues can cause, can lead to the knock-on effects of making us feel low and irritable. The physical symptoms of vaginal dryness and pain during sex can lead to loss of libido, anxiety and low mood.

Stressors in life – Stress can show up at any time in our lives, but there may be a number of factors that tend to coincide with the age of menopause for many women. During midlife, we may be faced with changes in our relationships and family structure. If we have children, they may still be young, or teenagers, or grown and left home, rendering us an 'empty nest'. Or we may have adult children still at home and be troubled by their stresses too. There may be issues related to work causing us stress, such as the demands of day-to-day tasks or concerns about organisational changes or thoughts about the prospect of retirement. This is also the age when our parents may be hitting a vulnerable stage in their lives with illness or reduced mobility/independence and so we may have to take on more of a caregiving responsibility, a well-known risk factor for depression.[19] Although these factors do not likely cause depression on their own, when we add menopausal symptoms to the mix, it can be harder to manage and potentially lead to depression. I think it is fair to say that menopause can be a time of significant life changes, and these can play a role in low mood or depression, depending on what they mean for us.

Menopause and neurodiversity

An area that has been little explored is how neurodiversity might impact on the menopausal experience. Neurodiversity refers to the different ways that our brain functions, learns and processes information, which has an impact on our behaviour, mood and social interaction. It is estimated that around one in seven people (more than 15% of the people in the UK) are neurodivergent.[20] This means their way of thinking, learning and processing is different to what is expected or considered the norm in society, that is, it is not neurotypical. There are a range of conditions that fall under the category of neurodivergence, including autism and attention deficit hyperactivity disorder (ADHD).

There is very limited research on autistic women's experience of menopause, so we have minimal knowledge on how autistic women navigate the menopausal transition and whether they experience additional challenges than those faced by their neurotypical counterparts. It is suggested that during perimenopause, autistic women might find that their pre-existing presenting symptoms of difficulties with sensory processing, emotion regulation, executive functioning and social interaction may be exacerbated. They may also experience new cognitive, social, emotional and sensory difficulties.[21] The National Autistic Society has produced a helpful guide to increase awareness of autism and menopause (see Resources).

Similarly, it is suggested that women with ADHD are more vulnerable to cognitive symptoms during menopause. When oestrogen levels drop during menopause, the levels of dopamine, the neurotransmitter essential for executive functioning, also reduces. For women with ADHD who already struggle with impaired executive functioning, this reduction in dopamine levels can result in severe cognitive dysfunction.[22]

My meno moments

I sometimes find that people think that as a psychologist I don't experience the same emotional ups and downs as they do or that I find it easier to deal with difficulties when they arise. I am often seen as the 'the strong one' in family and social circles. While it may be true that psychologists are more aware of their emotional reactions and more knowledgeable on ways to cope than lay-people, it is certainly not the case that we are immune to the emotions, pains and hardships that everyone else experiences. And we too can be caught out by our feelings. Also, being aware of coping strategies does not mean that we always practise them. This means that we can relate to the struggles just like everyone else and fluctuate in our ability to cope with difficulties.

- *Anxiety* – Of course, the Covid-19 pandemic was a difficult time for everyone and it turned our world upside down. I found it a particularly difficult time with respect to my perimenopausal symptoms. I doubt if many of us relished the idea of wearing a mask when they became recommended or compulsory. Having a tendency towards claustrophobia and wearing glasses, I found it even more of a dreaded prospect. Added to that, the sudden onslaught of a hot flush, just made being in any enclosed space, such as the underground or the local supermarket, difficult to bear. My glasses would steam up; I would steam up. And I would feel like I might faint. So, of course I did what most people do as a coping behaviour in unpleasant, anxiety provoking situations – I avoided going to such places if it meant I would have to wear a mask. As a psychologist, I was conscious of not allowing this to generalise to anxiety in more and more situations, and I gradually got back to normal after the mask-wearing rule was lifted.
- *Mood swings, low mood and irritability* – Now, I would like to say that I was this incredibly calm, zen-like person and then menopause came along and changed me. The truth is that although most of the time I am calm and 'together', I have been known to be fairly outspoken when in my comfort zone and can be quite impatient. That might sound contradictory to being a therapist, but in my therapist role I believe I have always been patient with my clients – I think that's because I don't have any expectations from them as I do of myself and those close to me. During my early perimenopausal years, when I was going through particularly bad symptoms, I started noticing that I became easily irritated by people and even less likely to hold back on letting them know. Maybe this is the confidence that comes with age, or maybe with all the mayhem of menopause, you really don't have time for 'nonsense' from others. I do

believe my developing spirituality has helped me mellow and become more patient in recent years.

- I generally tend to be in good spirits. But on the days when my joints are stiff and I have niggling pain in my knees and sharp pain in my thumb-joints, I can get quite low. And if I haven't slept very well the night before, I can feel tired and just worn down. On occasions, this may have the knock-on effect of impatience and irritability towards my family and perhaps even colleagues.
- I don't come from a 'sweary' family, and although growing up in London I heard expletives being used all the time, I don't think I said the word 'f***' out loud until well into my 40s. And to this day, I have never said it in front of my older brother or parents. But around the time when perimenopause hit, phrases like, 'what the f***!', 'f*** that!' and 'f*** off' became a part of my vocabulary, although *mostly*, this would be in my head or under my breath. Whereas, before I might have been disapproving about the use of expletives, I developed a new-found appreciation of their cathartic power and do not begrudge anyone using them. I would prescribe a mild and measured dosage of 'use as and when necessary'.
- It is also the relentless nature of this whole menopause journey that can wear you down. A recent episode of feeling low for me was the sudden appearance of my period after eight months of not having any bleeding at all. I thought I was on the home stretch, only four more months to go and I could declare myself as having reached menopause. But no, Auntie Meno decided to throw me a curve ball, just as I was getting into a good diet and exercise routine. And again, when I am on holiday. This time. I had become so confident that I would not have another period, I had not even brought any sanitary products. We were staying on a remote farm, so it was not as if I could just pop down to the nearest chemist. I had to go and explain the situation to the landlady, who appeared older than me and understood, so we had an interesting chat about menopause. Fortunately, she was able to get me what I needed from her adult daughter's bathroom. This incident led me to feel down for a few days, like I was fighting a losing battle. I'll tell you how I dealt with this in the next chapter.

Key points

Hormonal fluctuations and midlife stress can play havoc with our mental heath

We are significantly more vulnerable to depression during perimenopause than before

Doctors need to assess underlying causes for depression before deciding on the treatment approach

Today I am grateful for:

No longer needing to wear a mask when I go to the supermarket

Kind people who help have helped me out when in a predicament

My family, for being there through my mood shifts

Your turn:

List your **key learning points** from this chapter

List two or three things (big or small) you are **grateful for** right now

6 Coping with Stress, Anxiety and Worry

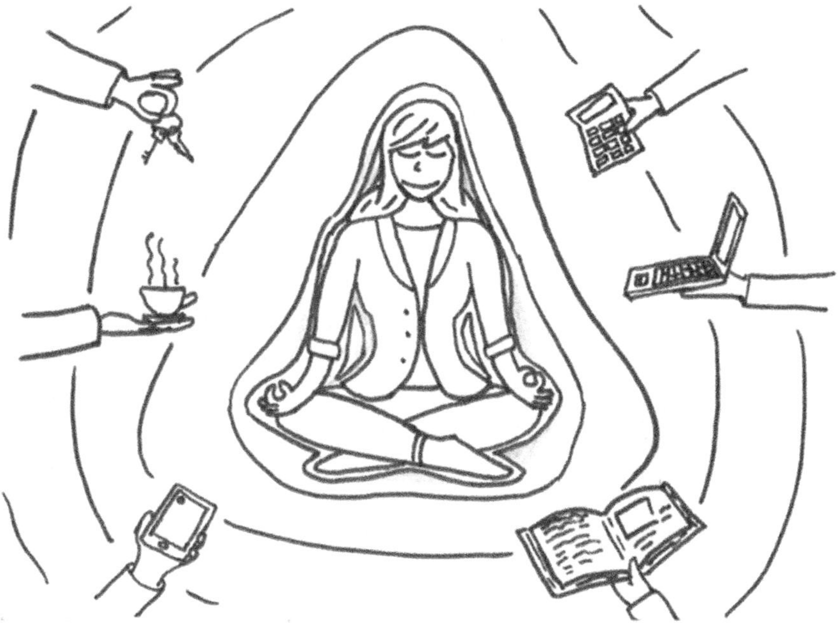

By learning about how our thoughts and behaviour are linked and how unhelpful patterns in these can play a role in causing and maintaining emotional distress, we can find ways to make changes that will help us live a less stressful life and minimise anxiety and distress. The changes I refer to here include shifting our perspective so that we learn to tolerate difficult emotions and establish a more positive outlook. The aim is to make the experience of menopause, among everything else that might be going on in our life, feel within our capacity to manage rather than feeling like an insurmountable burden.

Breaking the cycle of anxiety

Our anxiety state can manifest itself as physical sensations in our body, our interpretative thoughts about the situation, our emotional reactions and the way we react to it. All anxiety is related to fear in response to some form of threat. Biologically, we have a natural in-built response to anxiety or stress – our fight or flight response (the stress response discussed in Chapter 5) – which is a survival mechanism to protect us from actual danger. When appropriately triggered, this response can help us to cope with extreme situations and rise to many challenges. But the problem is that these days we get anxious about things that we *believe* to be threatening, such as making mistakes, losing control or embarrassing ourselves, rather than an actual danger, like a wild animal chasing us. Our anxiety may be based on an actual past negative experience in a similar situation or it might just be a general sense that something will go wrong.

When we start thinking something will go wrong or we won't cope, we set off the natural stress response. Our heart rate increases and we might have palpitations; we breathe faster and shallower causing us to feel shortness of breath or lightheadedness; we might feel our chest tightening; we might feel sweaty, shaky, nauseous; our muscles might feel tense, among other possible physical reactions. When we notice this happening in our body, we have what are called catastrophic interpretations – 'I'm having a heart attack'; 'I'm going to faint'; 'I'm going to embarrass myself'. So, then we try to do something to stop feeling like this. Our first instinct is usually to get out of the situation, to escape if we can – the flight response. If we can't escape, we try to find other forms of 'safety' or reassurance – we might sit down or ask someone for reassurance that everything is OK. And because these safety behaviours helped in that moment, we might start relying on them, thinking they made the anxiety go away, then get anxious if we can't do these things. Or we might avoid getting ourselves into such anxiety-provoking situations altogether in the future, so we don't have to deal with them at all – this is called avoidance. This whole process is described as a vicious cycle of anxiety, as shown in Figure 6.1.

This diagram uses the CBT approach to understanding the links between our thoughts, feeling and behaviours as reactions to a situation. It shows how the way we view the experience can be unhelpful and lead to negative feelings and unhelpful behaviours such as avoidance. We often think of avoidance as an effective way of coping with situations that make us uneasy or distressed, and we all use it to some extent. It does work in the short term because of course, if we keep ourselves away from a situation, we are not going to experience the unpleasant way it makes us feel. But in the long term, it can lead to further problems. If we keep avoiding things, we become more and more anxious about it. And by not facing it, we never find out that things might not be as we anticipate. Also, there are some situations that we can't actually avoid, such as a work meeting. So, how do we cope then?

In order to deal effectively with anxiety, we need to break the vicious cycle or reverse it. We need to face our fear and tackle the unhelpful thoughts and

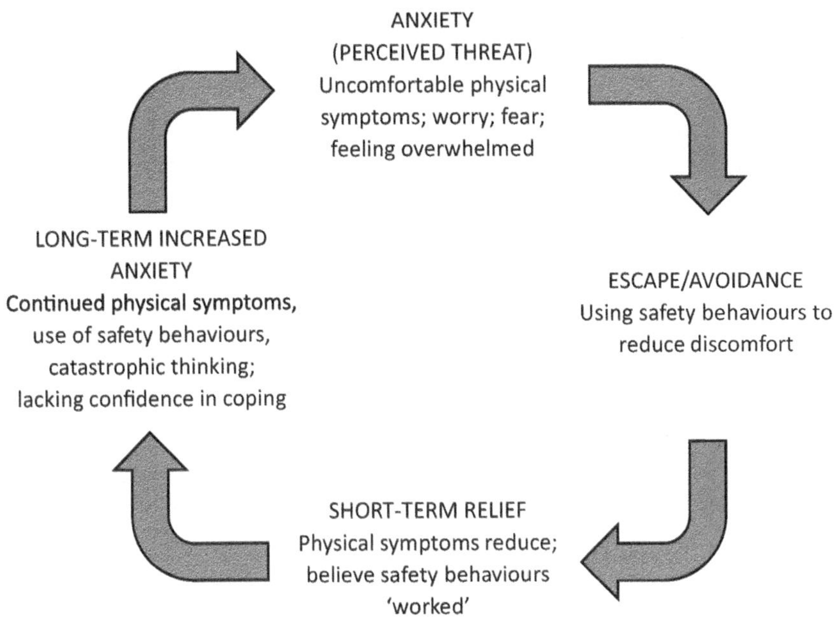

FIGURE 6.1 Vicious Cycle of Anxiety

behaviours. We need to stop avoiding and actually stay in the anxiety-provoking situation. If we are very anxious about something, just the thought of that will make us anxious. And when we do build up the courage to face the situation, it will initially make us feel the physical sensations of anxiety. But we can use techniques to help with that, such as breathing and relaxation exercises (see below).

Using these techniques, we can firstly calm our body, which will then enable us to think more clearly. We will not have such catastrophic thoughts and will be able to put things into perspective. This breaks the cycle and reduces our anxiety. We will discover what we don't find out if we avoid or escape the situation – that the anxiety does not keep rising but actually subsides and we really can cope. Of course, the first time of doing this will be hard, but once we do it, it will feel good and motivate us to try again. Once we've done it a few times, our confidence will improve and gradually over time, we will stop being so anxious. We will stop avoiding and might even end up forgetting what we were so anxious about. The coping cycle of anxiety in Figure 6.2 shows what it can look like when we have broken or reversed the vicious cycle and found a way to manage our anxiety.

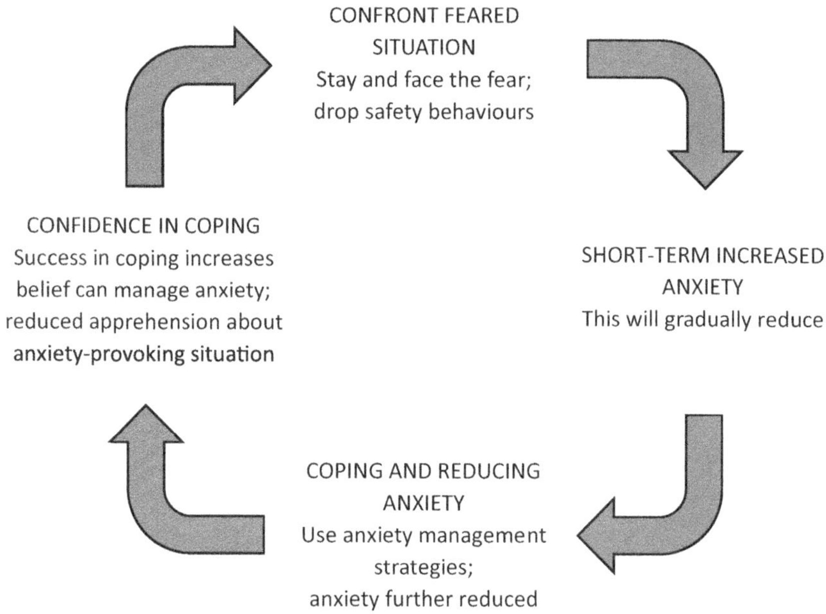

FIGURE 6.2 Coping Cycle of Anxiety

Breathing exercises

The first step to managing the physical experience of anxiety is to learn to regulate our breathing. When we are anxious, our breathing tends to be fast, irregular and shallow, a bit like the panting of a dog. Shallow breathing does not allow the diaphragm to work to its full capacity and restricts the lowest part of the lungs from getting the maximum amount of oxygenated air. This kind of breathing can leave us feeling short of breath, lightheaded and anxious that we will run out of breath, sometimes leading to panic as we think we might pass out. So, what we need to do is to regulate our breathing and practise a deeper, more paced way of breathing. When we breathe deeply, the diaphragm contracts more and enables the lungs to be fully filled with air and we get the maximum amount of air coming in and going out. This type of breathing can slow down our heartbeat and lower or stabilize our blood pressure. Deep breathing exercises can help us calm down, offsetting the physical symptoms of anxiety and prevent it from escalating into panic. Those of us used to doing sports, dance or yoga, are likely to already know such breathing exercises. They may be called diaphragmatic breathing, abdominal breathing, belly breathing, or paced breathing.

Here is a diaphragmatic breathing exercise I do myself and regularly show my clients:

- *Place one hand on your diaphragm (just below your chest and above your stomach) and the other on your chest.*
- *Now take a deep breath in through your nose so that you can feel your stomach lifting.*
- *Hold your breath to the count of four.*
- *Exhale slowly through your mouth to a count of six – you will feel your stomach dropping back down.*
- *Keep the hand on your chest as still as possible. If you notice your chest rising when breathing, try to concentrate more on drawing the air in, as if you are inflating a balloon in your abdomen.*

You might find it easier to do this lying down when you are first learning the technique – lie on your back on a flat surface or on a bed, with your knees bent and your head supported. You can use a pillow under your knees to support your legs. Subsequently, you will probably find it more convenient to do it in sitting positions – sit comfortably, with your knees bent and your shoulders, head and neck relaxed.

It will require regular practise, so it's best to do the exercise two to three times a day for a while until you are comfortable with it. It is best to practise when you are *not* anxious rather than trying it for the first time when in an anxious state. You could make it part of your daily routine by practising it before or after brushing your teeth each morning and night, for example. Once you have established it as a practice, it is a tool you have for when you need it.

Relaxation exercises

When we are stressed, our muscles tense up, and this muscular tension can lead to unhelpful bodily feelings, such as headache, tightness in the chest and backache. These aches and pains can make us even more anxious and tense. Relaxation slows down the body's systems and 'switches off' the feelings of tension. So, in addition to managing our breathing, we can manage the physical sensations of anxiety by practicing body relaxation exercises. With all that is going on in our menopausal mind and body, it is crucial that we recharge ourselves in order to adapt to the changes. This can sound easier said than done on a busy day. If we remind ourselves that relaxation exercises help us cope better with our menopausal symptoms, it might help us to prioritise it.

Relaxation exercises are more than just 'chilling out' – they require a determined effort to make time for yourself and train yourself to fully relax and change your mindset. Again, there are different types of relaxation exercises. The one I like to use most often, and which my clients report being effective when we practise it in session, is called progressive muscle relaxation (PMR). Developed by Edmund Jacobson,[1] it is based on his finding that muscles can be relaxed by tensing and then releasing them. If we do this progressively through the muscle groups, it builds a sense of deep relaxation in the whole body and promotes mental relaxation and better sleep.[2] To practise PMR, allow yourself 15 minutes in an undisturbed space. You can do it either sitting or lying down, preferably with your eyes closed –you could make a recording of the script below and play it back, or you can fnd a video on YouTube, such as the one by Therapist Aid. Try to notice how it feels each time you tense and relax your muscles.

- *Get into a comfortable position. Relax your body. Take a few deep, slow breaths.*
- *Clench your fists and hold them tight – count to 5 – release – count to 10.*
- *Draw your forearms towards your shoulders, fists closed, to tighten your biceps – hold the tension – count to 5 – release – count to 10.*
- *Straighten your arms in front of you, fists closed, and tense the muscles in the back of your arms – count to 5 – release – count to 10.*
- *Shrug your shoulders as high as you can – hold there for 5 – release – count to 10.*
- *Keeping your eyes close, open your mouth as far as it will go – hold the tension for 5 – release – count to 10.*
- *Press your tongue against the roof of your mouth and clench your jaw muscles – hold for 10 – release.*
- *Scrunch up your face, lips together, eyes shut tight, nose and forehead wrinkled – hold it all tense for 5 – release – count to 10.*
- *Tighten the muscles of your chest, stomach and abdomen, drawing them all in tensely – hold for 5 – release – count to 10.*
- *Gently press your neck back and gently arch up your lower back – hold for 5 – release – count to 10.*
- *Bring your head forward to your chest – hold for 5 – release – count to 10.*
- *Tense the muscles of your thighs by straightening your legs and pointing your toes forwards – hold for 5 – release – count to 10.*
- *Clench your buttocks, tense the back of your legs by straightening them and pointing your toes up to the ceiling – hold for 5 – release – count to 10.*
- *Curl your toes – hold tightly for 5 – release – count to 10.*
- *Your whole body should feel relaxed now. Allow yourself to enjoy this feeling for a few minutes, then count backwards from 10 to 1 as you gradually open your eyes.*

You should not be holding your breath during this practice. If you feel any discomfort or cramp while tensing any muscle, reduce the contraction or stop and move on to the next muscle. And don't worry too much about the order of things; it doesn't matter if you miss a muscle or change the order a bit.

The ability to relax doesn't always come naturally; it is a skill which has to be learned. So, this exercise will require some practise for you to feel the benefits over time. Set yourself a time to practise, as you are more likely to get into a routine which you can stick to. With consistent practise, you will become more aware of your muscles, how they respond with tension, and how you can relax them. Over time, you will train your body to respond differently to stress and anxiety.

Practicing mindfulness

The concept of mindfulness is thought to date back to around 2500 years in ancient Eastern and Buddhist philosophy though there is some form of mindfulness practised in other religions too. It is said to have been introduced to the Western world by Thich Nhat Hanh in the 1960s and 1970s when Buddhism and Eastern spirituality was very popular in USA. In 1979, Jon Kabat-Zinn separated mindfulness from the cultural, religious, and ideological principles of its past, making it more amenable to the 'Western mind' and culture, leading to the first formalised mindfulness-based intervention called Mindfulness-Based Stress Reduction (MBSR).[3] Since then, there has been substantial research showing how mindfulness improves mental health, so it has been widely accepted as an effective mental health self-management tool.[4]

Being mindful essentially requires you to just *be* – fully connecting with the 'now' moment, acknowledging and accepting your current thoughts and feelings, without judgement. Mindfulness exercises help you to train your brain to be still and relaxes your body too. Research with menopausal women has shown that mindfulness practise can alleviate anxiety symptoms[5] and is effective in the prevention of depressive symptoms during the menopausal transition.[6]

There are so many ways of practicing mindfulness. It can be practised as a meditation or you can do everyday activities, like breathing, walking, eating, and showering in a mindful way. You need to focus completely on the activity you are engaged in and use all your senses to fully experience the present moment and stay in it. If you find yourself drifting off into thoughts about the past or future, you practise noticing that and bringing your attention back to the mindfulness activity. There are many online resources available for practising mindfulness. One of my favourites to do is this mindful eating of an easy-peel clementine orange:[7]

- *Hold the orange in your hand and really look at it, like it's the first time you've seen one. Without making any judgements, describe the colour (what shade of orange is it?), shape and size.*
- *Move it around in your hand – how does it feel on your fingertips? What's the texture like? Is it cool or warm?*
- *Put it up to your nose and smell it – does it smell sweet or bitter? Is it a strong or faint smell?*
- *Slowly peel the orange – What do you notice? Is there a sound? What is revealed under the peel? Are there different textures? Does it smell stronger? Do you get juice on your fingers? How does that feel?*
- *Take a segment of the orange and observe it in the same way you did the whole orange. Slowly bring the segment to your mouth; notice how your mouth begins to water. Gently place it in your mouth, letting it lie on your tongue first – What does it feel like? Bite into it – what does it taste like? What sensations are you getting in your mouth? As you swallow it, what sensations do you notice in your throat as it goes down?*
- *You can take 10 minutes eating the orange, slowly appreciating every step and have a sensory moment of mindfulness, just you and your orange.*

Managing unhelpful thoughts

Our thoughts can be extremely powerful, and often we are not aware of the negative automatic thoughts we are having. As we have seen from the vicious cycle example, negative or unhelpful thoughts, can set off a chain of events which makes our anxiety worse, usually increasing the intensity of our body's responses. Within CBT, we use techniques that help us become aware of, actively challenge, and change our negative thinking patterns to more helpful or 'adaptive' ones. Within acceptance and commitment therapy (ACT), we talk about getting 'fused with' or 'hooked by' our difficult thoughts and feelings. Imagine yourself being picked up on the end of a fishing reel, being reeled in and swinging around all over the place as you become more and more caught up. Getting hooked in this way may make you act out in unhealthy ways or draw your focus away from what you are doing and more towards your negative thoughts. So, in ACT, we use 'cognitive defusion' techniques to change how we respond to negative thoughts rather than modify their content.

Here are a few such ACT and CBT techniques you can try to break a vicious cycle, or 'unhook' yourself from your difficult thoughts:

Thought defusion – This is a technique that helps to reduce the negative impact of thoughts. Firstly, notice the thought or feeling you are experiencing. Name it, either in your head or out loud. This helps to externalise it and distance yourself from the thought. For example, during a hot flush, you might say out loud, 'I'm having the thought that everyone will notice I'm sweating'. Then to distance yourself even further from that thought, you could add, 'I notice that I'm having the thought that everyone will notice I'm sweating'. It might seem an odd thing to do at first, but with practise you will find it will reduce the power of your thoughts, and the anxiety related to it will dissipate.

Thoughts on train metaphor – There are many ACT metaphors that can help you defuse from negative thoughts. I often use this one: imagine your negative thoughts are on a train and you are waiting on the platform as it comes in. You can choose to either jump onto the train and get 'hooked' by the thoughts or you can just let that train pass without jumping on. This might be difficult to do at first, but with practise, can help you become an observer of your mind's activity and enable you to spot when your mind is focusing on things that are unhelpful.

Putting things into perspective – This means taking a step back and looking at the situation from a wider context. Remember, anxious thoughts are not facts, they are just your view of a situation. Ask yourself whether the thought is actually true and whether there is any evidence for it. If you can't find any evidence for it, ask yourself why you should believe in this thought at all.

Challenging unhelpful thoughts – There are a number of questions you can ask yourself to help you challenge the thought and come up with alternative perspectives, such as:

- *Is this thought true? What are the facts? Or is it just my opinion?*
- *Is it helpful or useful to think this? Is this an old story – something I've told myself before?*
- *How might someone I think of as a calm and measured person respond in the same situation?*
- *What would I advise a loved one who is in a similar situation?*

Managing worries

If you find you worry all the time about lots of things, it can be quite exhausting. Here are a couple of techniques to try to cope with ongoing worries.

Set a worry time – One way to feel more in control is to contain your worries to within a short period of time in the day (your 'worry time'). Every time a worry pops up, tell yourself you will think about it in the worry time and use a mindfulness technique to let it go (see below). When the worry time comes, you will often find you have forgotten half the things you worried about as they were not that important. And for the worries that have persisted, you can either try and problem solve them (see Chapter 9) or let them go too.

Letting go of worries When we are worried by 'what if' thoughts about the future – such as 'what if I go blank when asked a question?'; 'what if I miss my alarm after not sleeping well tonight?' – they tend to fuel the vicious cycle of anxiety. If we take a closer look at what these worries are, we can ask ourselves how realistic/likely or unlikely they are to happen. If they are actual things that could happen, we can think about how we might tackle them, taking a problem-solving perspective and making a plan of action (discussed further in Chapter 9). If we decide they are very unlikely, we need to weigh up whether they are worth the anxiety they are causing. We often realise they are not worth it, but don't know how to let them go. You could try this cloud metaphor mindfulness technique:[8]

> *Think about your most recent worry. What was the triggering thought? Bring that thought into your mind. Imagine your thought is like the clouds – you would not try to control the clouds – you would just allow them to exist in their own space, knowing they will eventually pass you by. Similarly, watch your thought and do nothing to control it or influence it in any way. Just watch the clouds. You may notice that they are moving, but don't make them move. You may notice the thought fades, but don't make it fade. You may notice other thoughts come and go – let them. Just watch the thought in a detached way. Like the clouds, it will soon pass.*

Accepting that not everything is in your control – My spiritual approach to managing anxiety and letting go is through prayer. I see prayer as a way of entrusting my fears to a higher being (God) with the faith that He will help me through difficult situations. So, once I have 'handed over' my worries, I can let go of them, and this, in turn, reduces my anxiety. Again, it is easier said than done at times. It requires reminders and practise. And it does not mean that I take no responsibility for my thoughts and take no action when it is within my capacity to resolve issues or help myself. I still have to do my bit in trying to manage with the tools available to me. But I also accept that the ultimate outcome is not within my control, so there is no point in fretting over it. To give a practical example, when I leave my car parked somewhere, I have a responsibility to lock it. Having done that, I can safely walk away with the expectation that it will be there when I get back. If I come back to find my car has been stolen, that was outside of my control. If I had spent all my time worrying 'what if my car gets stolen', I could not have prevented the theft and the ruminating would only have ruined my experience of whatever I was doing. So even if I pray, I still have to take the necessary action to secure my property.

The prayer gives me a second level of confidence that I am being backed up by a powerful force.

Re-evaluating your load and shedding perfectionism

If you actually have a lot on your shoulders, the self-management approaches described above are not going to be enough. You can't wish away all the chores and responsibilities. But you also cannot just carry on – if some things are weighing you down for a long time, they will eventually become too much to manage. So, you might need to take stock of what is *really* necessary for you to do, what might be shared with others, what is important to you and what are the less important things you could let go off. Assessing how much of a burden everything is and thinking about how it all fits in with your values will help you make decisions about what needs to change. You can also think about whether some tasks can be set aside for a later time, or whether some burdens can be shared with others. This will enable you to be left with only what you can comfortably manage.

This may be where perfectionism comes in. Are you someone who is getting anxious trying to achieve the high standards you set yourself? There is nothing wrong with expecting yourself to do well. But ask yourself how realistic those expectations are. Are you constantly setting yourself up for failure? What is driving these expectations? Do they fit in with your own values? (see Chapter 8 for developing meaningful goals).

Non-attachment

If can be beneficial to develop a perspective in life that nothing is permanent – nothing remains exactly the same, everything changes, and everything passes. It helps by not letting us get too attached to things (material or otherwise) and makes it easier to let things go and move on.

My faith teaches me to not hold anything in this world too dearly, and difficult as that is to accept, it provides a sense of freedom. It makes it easier to let go of things. To not worry about small things for a start, but not even about bigger things. For example, being brought up by an over-protective mother, I realised that I am prone to being over-protective towards my own children. But when I remind myself of the principle that they are not 'mine', but simply blessings within this world that I am passing through, I can give myself permission to let go and give them the freedom to make their own choices in life. This, then, reduces my anxiety and stress about always needing to be in charge of things.

In a similar vein, it helps to remind ourselves that our existence on this earth is transitory. Until there are huge advances in science to preserve life, none of us are here forever. And we can't take anything with us when we die. If you visit a cemetery and read the headstones, you will see that people die at any age and leave behind people who care about them. Now this might sound like a morbid thing to do, but in fact it can be quite a positive experience. By reminding us of our own mortality, it can motivate us to make the most of life, doing things we value and spending time with those most precious to us. It can make worldly desires like wealth and power seem less important, thus reducing stress and anxiety about them – what Alain de Botton refers to as 'status anxiety'[9].

Key points

When anxious, think of the vicious cycle and how you can break it

Breathing and relaxation exercises take practise – make time in your day for these useful tools

There are numerous ways of effectively challenging unhelpful thoughts

Today I am grateful for:

Breathing and relaxation exercises

My reminders and ongoing practise of trying not to hold things in this world too dearly

Having achieved a slower pace of life over the past few years

Your turn:

List your **key learning points** from this chapter

List two or three things (big or small) you are **grateful for** right now

7 Mood Management

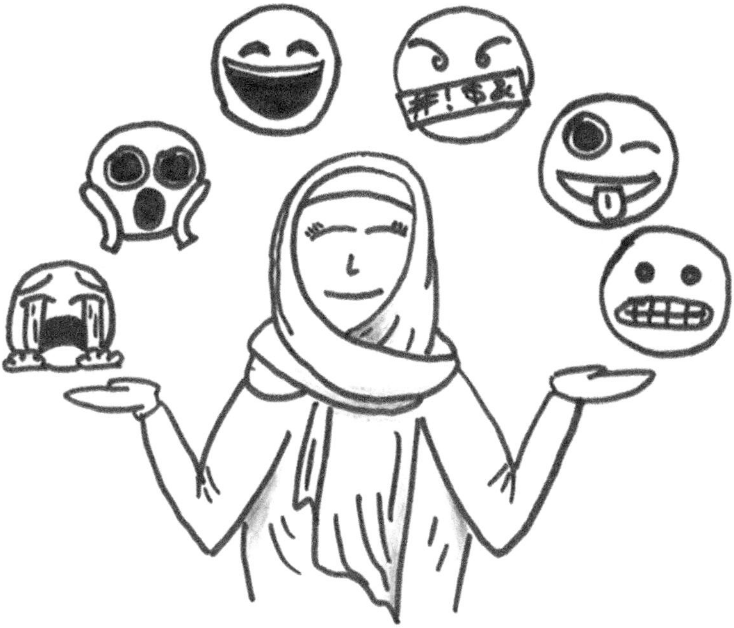

Becoming aware of our moods

We don't often stop and reflect on how exactly it is we are feeling in a situation. Sometimes we just go about things in a sort of automatic motion and don't 'catch up' with ourselves until we are really distressed. Then we can't work out how we got there. Sometimes, we just know we don't feel right, but can't quite put our finger on what it is that is bothering us or don't know the words to describe it. But if we check in on ourselves now and then, and especially when we notice a shift in mood, we can learn to start paying attention to, and picking up on, how we are feeling. You could do a little exercise right now and see how many words you can think of to describe your feelings in this moment.

Noticing[1] – This is a technique for tuning in to yourself and can help you pick up on how you are reacting to different situations. To observe what is going on for you, you need to tune in to your mind and body. It is important to use your bodily senses to only observe, and not apply any judgement or self-criticism. You can try these things to notice your actions, thoughts and feelings:

- *Take a few deep breaths, slow down what you are doing and 'watch' yourself – notice what you are doing as you are doing it.*
- *Observe your posture – how you are carrying yourself in terms of your posture and where you are placing your hands. You don't need to change anything, just notice.*
- *Gently check in on your body – Are there any areas where you feel tense, stiff or any pain? You don't have to deal with it now as you are just noticing.*
- *When a thought, image or memory comes into your mind, acknowledge it, don't try to push it away, but don't get caught up in it either – just let it pass.*
- *You can also build your practice of noticing by observing outside of yourself. For example, you could go to the park and notice the trees, birds, other people and animals. Try pretending you are an alien who has just landed on earth so it is the first time you are experiencing these things.*

Try to do these noticing activities for at least a few minutes. If you find that your mind wanders and you lose focus, that's OK. Gently bring your focus back to noticing. The more you practise, the better you will get at noticing and being in touch with yourself.

Mood tracking or journaling

As we have seen, it is common to experience unexpected shifts in mood, as well as episodes of depression, during the menopausal years. If frequent and/or unexpected mood changes are particularly problematic for you during your menopausal journey, tracking your mood is a good tool to use. The aim of doing this is to help you regulate your moods so that you minimise unexpected shifts in mood which can take you by surprise and cause upset. You might also want to record your anxiety, irritability, anger and other emotions.

By charting your mood at regular intervals, you can:

- look for patterns in how your mood changes over time
- consider if certain situations or circumstances might be triggering it – what are the warning signs? can they be avoided?
- observe any impacts from factors such as your diet, daily activities and sleep on your mood
- work out which coping strategies you try are effective in improving your mood

There are so many ways you can do this. See Table 7.1 for an example you can use or adapt to suit what you want to record.

Ideally, you could try and record your mood at regular intervals during the day – say morning, early afternoon and in the evening – to get a picture of how it fluctuates throughout the course of the day. However, if this seems too onerous a task, at least a check-in with yourself once a day (but not exactly the same time each day) could still be useful. Table 7.1 provides a template for recording twice a day. Also, remember you are not just focusing on negative moods. To get an idea of how your mood fluctuates, you need to record the ups as well as the downs at the selected time of recording. That's how you can then differentiate what makes for good moods and what leads to low moods.

Alternatively, you may prefer a less structured way to track your mood, such as keeping a journal in a notebook or notes in your phone. For me, writing down my thoughts and reflections comes quite naturally. However, over the years, time became an issue, so I'd often start writing in notebooks but not completing my notes and not getting around to filling in the blank spaces I had left. That's what led to my 'meno moments' notes on my phone as a briefer journaling approach to keeping track of my symptoms, moods and thoughts, even before the idea of writing this book came about. There are also mobile apps available for journaling purposes if you prefer.

Getting outdoors

We will discuss in the next chapter how important exercise is to our general wellbeing. And even better for us is to do exercise or other activities outdoors. Being out in the sunshine gives us a boost of vitamin D which not only helps absorb the calcium that is necessary for bone health, but has also been shown to play an important role in regulating serotonin and melatonin, both of which are good for our mental health, especially for mood and sleep.[2] Getting out into nature – for example, a walk in the park, joining a forest-bathing group, or simply spending time in the garden – has been shown to have a restorative effect on our mind and body.[3]

Doing it anyway!

Often when we are feeling low, we lack motivation and tell ourselves that we will wait until we are in a better mood before doing anything active. How long will we wait? And how will that happen? Something has to set things into motion. So, we actually need to turn that idea on its head and realise that rather than waiting to be in the mood, we need to just take the action even when we don't feel like it and that in itself will improve our mood and motivate us. For example, on a miserable

Weekly Mood Tracker

MOOD	Monday		Tuesday		Wednesday		Thursday		Friday		Saturday		Sunday	
	am	pm	am	pm	am	pm	am	pm	am	pm	am	pm	am	pm
+3														
+2														
+1														
My normal														
-1														
-2														
-3														
Hours slept (previous night)														
Sleep quality (poor/OK/good)														
Medication														
Physical exercise														
Stressors (describe)														

In the mood section, select the box that best fits your mood rating, then in that box write a word to describe your mood. For example:

On Monday morning, if you feel worried and a little lower in mood than normal, you would write 'worried' in the -1 box for Mon am.
On Wednesday afternoon, if you're going to meet up with an old friend, you might put 'excited' in the +3 box for Wed pm.

You can give other descriptions of what's going on for you in the boxes for sleep, medication etc.

Here is a list of some words you might use to describe your mood, but of course you can use any words you want:

Happy – Calm – Excited – Pleased - Proud – Productive – Grateful – Content – Peaceful – Relaxed - Hopeful
Sad – Bored – Nervous – Angry – Irritated – Worried – Frustrated – Lonely – Stressed – Hurt – Ashamed

TABLE 7.1 Weekly Mood Tracker

autumnal morning or evening after work, we might not feel like going for a walk or to the gym and would rather stay cosy indoors. But if we force ourselves to do it anyway, we usually feel good and are glad we did it. Having a walking partner or a gym buddy can be helpful for encouraging each other when one or the other is not quite in the mood.

Fostering the attitude of gratitude

Gratitude is the recognition and acknowledgment of the good things in life and being appreciative of them. We generally tend to show appreciation for the bigger things – some profound event or experience – like graduating from university, having a baby or surviving an accident. And we often take for granted the small everyday things. These might be essential things like the availability of food, water and heating, our health and relationships, or even smaller pleasant things like the beauty of the nature around us. Developing an attitude of gratitude is about making a conscious habit of expressing appreciation on a regular basis, for the small things that we might usually take for granted, as well as the big. Even when we are really finding life difficult, consciously bringing our attention to things like the sun shining or having a laugh with a friend can help us to develop a more balanced perspective.

Having a grateful mindset can have positive effects across all aspects of our life. It helps us feel more optimistic, happier and satisfied with life.[4,5] It leads to higher self-esteem and valuing ourselves more positively, as well as being more compassionate towards ourselves and others.[6] Gratitude can make us feel more motivated, so we are more likely to work towards our goals and fulfil our ambitions. Research has shown that those with higher levels of gratitude are likely to have lower levels of depression.[7]

So, here are a few ways you can practise gratitude:

- *Count your blessings* – This is what I have tried to model for you with my gratitude box at the end of each chapter. At the end of the day – maybe after dinner or at bedtime – ask yourself, 'What am I grateful for today?' Try to think of three things, even the smallest of things that made you smile, feel good, or went right. Say them out loud. Even better, you could do this with others in your life as a shared exercise. With continued practice, you will find that you start noticing more positive things during your day.
- *Keep a gratitude journal* – Get into the habit of writing down the good things that have happened that day, no matter how small.
- *Acknowledge others' help and say thank you* – Show your appreciation to someone who has had an impact on your life verbally or in writing. This will nurture good relationships, which in turn will make you feel good. You can even appreciate someone mentally by thinking about how they helped you, thanking them in your mind, or praying for them.

- *Pray or meditate* – If you are spiritual, prayer can serve as a reminder to be thankful for what you appreciate. Or you can use mindfulness meditation – for example, noticing the sound of birds, the warmth of the sun and so on.

Developing self-compassion

We are often much better at showing kindness and compassion towards those that we care about, more so than to ourselves. We can often compare ourselves to others, even put ourselves down for not achieving what others have or what we expected of ourselves. We might be very self-critical, use harsh statements towards ourselves and beat ourselves up for decisions or actions we later regret. We would not normally be so judgemental towards those we love. So, what stops us having the same degree of kindness and compassion for ourselves that we are capable of having towards others? It may be a reflection of the way we have been treated ourselves in the past, and beliefs and habits we have built up over time. For example, if we were criticised by others, we might be more critical of ourselves and feel like we are never quite measuring up. Having a sense of low self-worth can make us believe we are not deserving of kindness.

The good news is that we can change these habits. Firstly, by noticing them, and acknowledging they are there. Then we can ask ourselves how helpful they are. Do we really get more out of ourselves when we are highly self-critical? If we think we do, is there a cost to treating ourselves this way? Or would it actually be kinder and less hurtful to say, 'Never mind, I'll try harder next time'? How do we feel when others praise us? Why not do that for ourselves when we do something well or make some improvement in an area of our life. If we're having an off day and nothing seems to be going right, why not just let things be for a while, then pick things up again slowly.

As an example, I'll describe how I practised self-compassion during my 'meno moment' incident I mentioned in the previous chapter – when I had a sudden return of bleeding after eight months. It was disappointing to say the least, as I was expecting to make it to 12 months, to reach what would be clinically defined as my point of menopause. I thought, 'I'm 54! It's not fair to still be bleeding when the average age of menopause is 51! AND I started my periods so early!' I remember reading somewhere a while back that a woman menstruates for an average of 40 years. If that was true, and I started my periods aged 10, it should all have been over for me a few years ago. But 'Auntie Flo' keeps turning up like a bad penny! I had got so used to not having periods. I did not miss them at all. Now having a period felt so cumbersome again – having to think about being prepared, carrying sanitary products and being careful to avoid leaks. Worse still was that the bleeding was so heavy, it felt like starting my periods all over again, and I was feeling drained like I did then. All this led to me feeling down for a few days. I felt like I was fighting a losing battle. I was not in the mood for following my diet and exercise plan – 'what was the point!'. I was also upset that I couldn't do my daily prayers on the prayer mat as this is not allowed when menstruating. It made me realise how I had got used to the routine of praying regularly without any breaks and found it so comforting and stabilising.

Then I made the conscious decision to show myself some compassion. I could ease off from my planned exercises for a few days and allow myself some comfort food too. I reminded myself that there was nothing to stop me adapting my prayers to alternative ones off the mat for a week. I allowed myself a couple of evenings of binge-watching a drama series on Netflix without feeling guilty that I should be doing something more productive. I reminded myself that I had been through this, and worse, many times before, and told myself to be patient as this too will pass. As my bleeding became lighter after a few days, I started picking up on my routines again.

Here is a reflective exercise to help you learn to be more compassionate towards yourself:

- *Think about some times when someone you care about told you that they are struggling with things or were feeling bad about themselves. Assuming you were feeling OK yourself at the time, how did you respond to them? What sort of things did you say? What tone did you speak in? How else did you comfort them – perhaps reaching out a hand or giving them a hug?*
- *Then think about some times when you were struggling or feeling bad about yourself. How did you respond to yourself during those times? What sort of things did you say to yourself? What tone did you use? Did you do anything to comfort yourself?*
- *Did you notice a difference between how you treat others and how you treat yourself? If so, why do you think that is? Why do you think you don't deserve the same treatment?*
- *Ask yourself how things might be different if you treated yourself the same way you treat someone you care about. Better still, practise doing it.*

Staying in touch with others

When you are not feeling at your best, it can seem easier to pull away from others and keep to yourself. You might do this for a number of reasons – you don't want people to see you at your worst; you are worried about being judged, being a burden or spoiling others' mood; you don't know how to talk about how you're feeling; you feel disconnected from others. However, isolation can make things worse. It can lead to unhealthy behaviours like drinking excessive alcohol and reduced activity, which can have knock-on effects on your health and loneliness. Loneliness has been shown to be a serious issue for people of all ages, especially in urban communities. I think the post-Covid practice of more people working from home and having less opportunities to socialise will only exacerbate this. It has been shown in a recent large scale research paper that social isolation and loneliness increase the risk of mortality, even for physically healthy people.[8] So, making healthy and supportive connections with others is important for our wellbeing. Try to notice when you are withdrawing – don't cancel those social plans and push yourself to connect by sending messages and calls and arranging walks and meet-ups with friends (see the section on 'positive human connections' in Chapter 8).

Opening up

A survey of 2,000 women in the UK who had experienced perimenopause found 8 out of 10 did not speak about the mental health issues they had experienced even with their partner or spouse.[9] Talking to others and sharing what is happening may come more easily to some of us than others. If we are influenced by an attitude of stigma towards ageing, menopause or mental health, we might not feel comfortable to open up to someone else about it. We might have past experiences of sharing that did not go well or messages from childhood to not show our vulnerability to others. Coming from a conservative family where these things are considered 'private matters', I did not initially find it easy to talk about my personal experience, even among female friends. And I still wouldn't talk about it with most family members. But my professional training is of course all about talking, so I am now very good at opening the dialogue and talking about my personal experience. I have found this to be a good source of support.

If you can overcome obstacles, such as I have just mentioned, opening up to selected others can have a number of benefits, such as:

- feeling validated when you express your feelings and experience
- picking up ideas about coping as you hear from other women who have navigated menopause, making it a good learning experience
- developing a bond through sharing

As to how you go about starting a conversation about personal or emotional issues, it will of course depend on your relationship with the other person. If you are not used to it, you could build up slowly weaving things into conversations and you will increasingly become more comfortable in opening up. You will gradually build up a support network which can be a source of comfort. If you do not have access to people within your own network, there are online forums and local support groups available (see the Further Support and Resources at the bac).

Seeking professional help

What I have described in this chapter are self-management approaches for coping with the psychological symptoms associated with menopause. If you find that your symptoms are too overwhelming to manage alone or are persisting after your efforts in using these approaches, consider seeking help from a qualified mental health professional. It may be that there are underlying issues which are also impacting or other factors in your life making it harder to cope. A counsellor, clinical psychologist, health psychologist or other professional in this field can help you talk through and understand what you are experiencing and support you in overcoming the issues. Your doctor would be the first person to consult – they may refer you to one of these professionals for talking therapy or signpost you to finding one. You should seek out someone registered with a professional and/or statutory body and check their credentials (see Resources).

There is further information on where to seek help for mental health problems in Further Support and Resources at the back.

Key points

Practise noticing your own moods

Be kind to yourself when things don't go as expected and grateful for what you do have/has gone well

Push yourself to get out and be active, and stay in touch with others to benefit from the connection

Today I am grateful for:

Realising that sometimes I have to push myself to do things rather than wait to be 'in the mood'

Having overcome my avoidance of talking about 'personal matters' and benefitting from sharing my experiences with friends

Your turn:

List your **key learning points** from this chapter

List two or three things (big or small) you are **grateful for** right now

8 Maintaining General Wellbeing

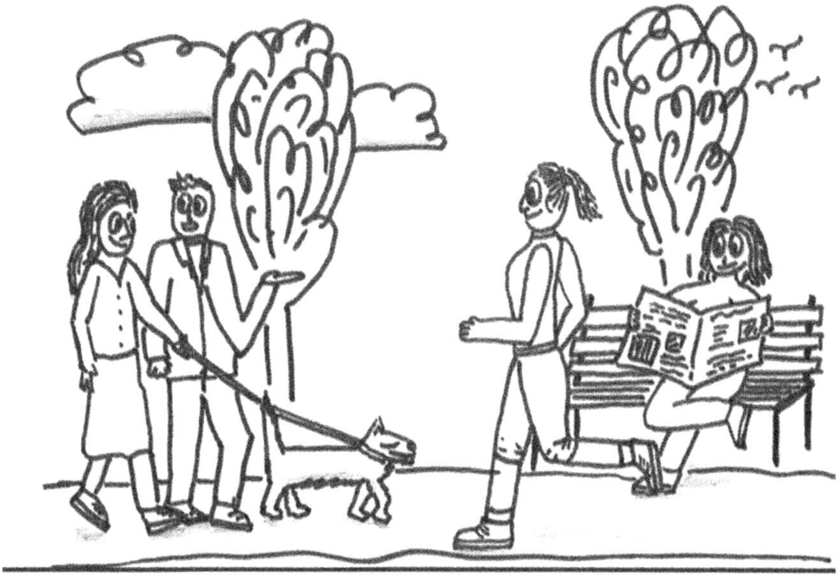

Taking care of ourselves is a crucial part of living well with menopause. That means keeping an eye on our physical health and dealing with any concerns as they arise, developing good habits, maintaining healthy relationships, and engaging in activities that keep us in good spirits. In essence, tending to the needs of the whole self. Some of the ideas I describe here will simply seem like 'common sense'. The thing is, there are many things we all know will benefit us, but we don't always act on them. For example, we have all been told enough times about eating our 'five-a-day' of fruit and vegetables for a healthy diet, but most of us struggle to stick to it.[1] So, we need reminders. We need to explore what stops us from putting into practice things that we know are good for us. What excuses do we make for ourselves? What unhelpful patterns have we got into? Identifying and understanding these obstacles will help us overcome them and enable us to start practising using tools that will help us. We also need to remember that if we have a go at something, and it doesn't quite lead to the result we were looking for, we have not failed, we just have to keep at it. Consistent practice is the key to reinforcing skills and developing good habits, helping us make steady progress toward healthy goals.

Overall healthy living

Establishing structure and routine

Having a sense of what to expect next grounds us and makes us feel secure. Establishing routines around our everyday essential activities like sleeping, eating, working and exercising helps us to structure our day and function to our optimal capacity. I would, however, always emphasise the need for some flexibility around this. If we are too rigid with our routines, it can create anxiety when things don't go completely to plan. We may also try to get a sense of 'control' driven by an inability to tolerate some degree of uncertainty. For some, routine may sound boring, so again it should not be so rigid that there is no room for spontaneity too. Often it is the spontaneous moments in life that bring us immense joy, so we don't want to lose that.

The importance of exercise

We all know the importance of keeping fit to maintain our health at any age. This is even more important during the menopausal transition. The recommendation for physical activity for adults aged 18–64 years given by the World Health Organisation (WHO) is:[2]

- At least 150 minutes of moderate-intensity physical activity (such as brisk walking or riding a bike) throughout the week, or at least 75 minutes of vigorous-intensity physical activity (such as walking up the stairs, running, swimming, cycling fast or uphill), or an equivalent combination of both.
- For additional health benefits, adults should increase their moderate-intensity physical activity to 300 minutes per week or equivalent.
- Muscle-strengthening activities should be done involving major muscle groups on two or more days a week

Exercise releases endorphins, which are the 'feel good' chemicals for the brain. So, getting some level of daily exercise will help your mood. During menopause, there are some exercises that are more helpful than others, as described in Chapter 12. If like me, you become aware that you are not as active as you should be, you might take the 'boom and bust' approach to exercise. I would get motivated to start exercising after a period of lethargy and decide to 'really get into it'. Then, I would inevitably overdo it – doing too much too quickly – and cause myself an injury, ironically leading my good intentions to become a period of inactivity as I couldn't exercise again until I had recovered. With that unhelpful approach, for someone who is not particularly sporty, I have acquired a few 'sports' injuries!

So, let's look at the healthier approach. If you have not done much exercise in a while, you should consult with your doctor about your plans. It is generally best to start with short periods of exercise and build up gradually and exercise regularly. To keep motivated, do exercises that you actually enjoy; it is important to do them at a level that you are comfortable with and slowly build up the intensity if you want, and the duration. Of course, any exercise is better than none, but if you can aim for at least 20–30 minutes of moderate exercise a day, on most days of the week, that should be beneficial.

Make your activities meaningful to you

Research has shown that although money or material things might make us happy to a certain extent,[3] we benefit more from a sense of purpose and meaningful activity. Such activity might be work or something else that motivates us and makes us feel happy or as I prefer to say, content. We feel good when we have a sense of achievement and enjoyment. And an even stronger factor in our contentment is when we feel a sense of connectedness to others, as found by the directors of the longest running scientific study of happiness.[4] This may be in the form of close relationships with family, friends, our community, or spiritual connectedness to a higher power. So, how do we decide what is meaningful to us? Well, we need to think about our values and what we can do to live more in line with what is important to us. (See the section on values below.)

Adopting a balanced lifestyle

One of the points that is consistently made when we research into management of health conditions and our physical and mental wellbeing in general is the importance of a healthy lifestyle. The WHO defines health as a 'state of complete physical, mental, and social wellbeing.'[5] This includes eating a balanced diet, regular exercise, getting adequate rest and maintaining optimal emotional health.

A healthy lifestyle is a balanced lifestyle. I often use this table analogy with my clients to demonstrate this point (I'm not entirely sure where it originates from, but the concepts are based on the behavioural activation model within CBT).[6] I start by asking how many legs a table needs. I am not asking here about pedestal tables with only one leg or designer three-legged tables, but rather a solid, bog-standard table – so 'four legs' is the answer I am looking for. Each leg corresponds to the things we need for a healthy, meaningful life – **P**hysical health; a sense of **A**chievement; a sense of **C**onnection; and a sense of **E**njoyment. The acronym PACE can be used as a reminder of the four components of a balanced life (see Figure 8.1).

This analogy can be further extended to consider what happens when we cannot achieve this balance, which can be the reality of life at times. For example, there may be phases when we have so many commitments, or we are physically unwell, that we struggle to find time to engage in enjoyable activities. The table would still be standing if one leg was a little weak for a while, but if you neglected it for too long, it might become shaky and not be able to hold its weight. And if you neglected two legs, the table is likely to collapse. So, we need to keep an eye on all four legs to keep it functioning as a good sturdy table.

So how do we achieve this healthy and balanced lifestyle? Often, we know what is required, but 'life' gets in the way. Or, we make an effort but struggle to keep it up, even if we have seen some positive gains. Achieving long-term behavioural change is rarely straightforward. But, if we keep re-committing to our goals and learning what can get in the way of us achieving them, we can make changes over time. Change doesn't happen overnight, but with consistent effort, we will start noticing improvements, so it is worth keeping up the momentum. Also, it is normal to have ebbs and flows in our motivation. So, if we go through a slow patch, we need to remember to be kind to ourselves (see discussion on self-compassion in Chapter 7). Then, when we are ready, we can re-set our goals and get back on track.

Adopting a balanced lifestyle is about bringing together all the factors we have mentioned above – a balanced diet, regular exercise, establishing structure and routine in our daily activities. Our activities should incorporate things that we enjoy, things that give us a sense of accomplishment and things that help connect us to

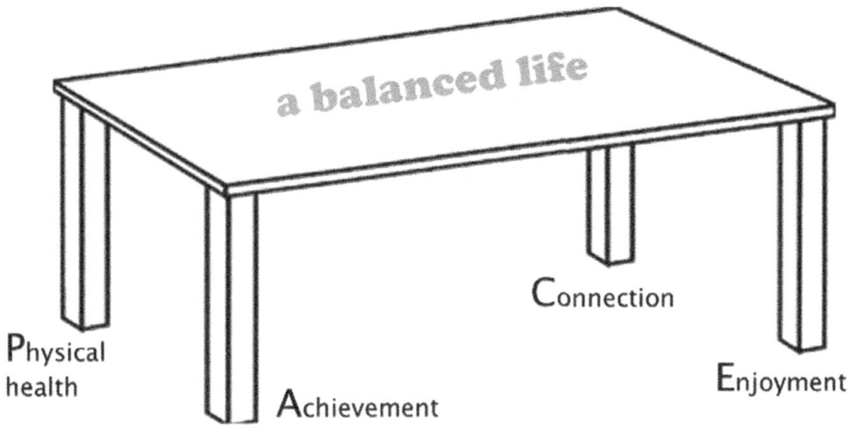

FIGURE 8.1 Tabe Analogy for a Balanced Life

others. Reading this list might be enough to put you off going any further! But you don't have to do this all at once; it's about taking a gradual approach. First, take stock of how you are currently doing in terms of the four pillars of a healthy lifestyle. This is your 'baseline' or starting point. Once you have identified which areas you need to work on, identify the order in which you want to tackle them, prioritising one area at a time. You might think your diet is not too bad right now, but you could do with exercising more, so you could make that your focus for a few months. Or perhaps you've been so busy with work and family, you haven't had a chance to catch up with friends, so you might make an extra effort to call one or two friends or arrange to meet up.

I have developed a Balanced Lifestyle Log (Table 8.1), which you can use as a template to get you started. I have completed one column with an example of one of my working days. For the first week, complete it as things are now. Remember to do the ratings of Achievement, Connection and Enjoyment (A-C-E), as this will help you see which activities lead to most contentment and will also help you identify where the 'gaps' are. Then start thinking about what is missing in terms of the range or quality of your activities and how you want to fill those gaps. Ask yourself questions like:

- *What did I use to enjoy and value that I haven't done for a while?*
- *What gives me a sense of purpose that I haven't felt for some time?*
- *Have I lost connection with people whose company I used to enjoy?*

Don't forget the 'P' leg of the balance table. Looking after your physical health includes being mindful of having a healthy diet, keeping up-to-date with health check-ups, and of course regular exercise. When you do exercise, it might be rated as an achievement and/or enjoyment and even connection if you are exercising with others. One tip for making you more likely to stick to exercise routines is to attach it to another activity you do daily – for example, you could go for a walk or run immediately after you finish work as a nice way of marking the end of the working day. For me, I like 'tea and Pointless' (a daily television quiz show) time with my husband around 5 p.m. on days we are both working from home. So, I do my daily walk at lunch time and my yoga or weight-training session after my sunset prayer and before dinner.

Once you have established your baseline, you can then work on increasing activities that will improve your ratings on A-C-E. It is also helpful to rate your mood at the end of each day, so you can see the impact of your daily activity and you can do more of what makes you feel good. Over time, you will have a healthy range of activities that are meaningful to you, and you will have developed a structured week with good routines, all serving to make you feel more balanced and content. This

Balanced Lifestyle Log

In each time slot (can change to suit you), make a brief note of your activity. Then rate these aspects in relation to the activity on a scale of 1-10 (1=least; 10 = most): Your sense of **Achievement** for the activity on a scale of 0-10 (A=?) your sense of **Connectedness** to others/higher power (C = ?), and your sense of **Enjoyment** (E = ?) from doing the activity. At the end of each day, rate your overall mood for that day (0 = lowest to 10 = highest).

Day / Time Period	Example	Monday	Tuesday	Wednesday	Thursday	Friday	Saturday	Sunday
7 – 9 am	Got up & shower (A=4) Breakfast alone (E = 6)							
9 - 11 am	Working at home - finished report due tomorrow (A=8; E=5)							
11am-1pm	Business meeting online (A=5; C=3; E=3)							
1pm - 2pm	Prayed (C=5) Lunch (E=5) Walked to clinic (E=5)							
2 - 4pm	Two client sessions in clinic (A=9; E=7)							
4 – 6pm	Walked home; picked up shopping (A=6); Tea & 'Pointless' (E=8)(C=7)							
6 - 8pm	Online yoga (A=8; E=8); Cooked (A=8;E=7) Prayed (C=7)							
8 - 10pm	Dinner with family (C=8); Mum's call(C=6); Prepared work for tomorrow (A=7)							
10pm – 12mn	Watched TV (E=6) Prayed (C=9); Went to bed by 12 (A=9)							
MOOD RATING	8							

TABLE 8.1 Balanced Lifestyle Log

approach does not mean you will be losing all spontaneity in your life – you can still allow some flexibility in your routine so that there is scope for incorporating new and varied activities.

Diet and nutrition

Eating a healthy and balanced diet is, of course, not a recommendation just for menopausal women, but for everyone throughout our lives. However, there are some foods which are thought to be particularly beneficial during the menopausal transition. It's been widely acknowledged for some time now that following a typical Mediterranean diet and lifestyle leads to significant reduction in the experience of menopausal symptoms. It is suggested that high fibre in this kind of diet can help stabilise oestrogen levels.[7] Neuroscientist, Dr Lisa Mosconi, explains in her book 'The XX Brain' why the Mediterranean diet is perfectly suited to women's health. She shares research evidence demonstrating why diet and nutrition is specifically important for our cognitive functioning during menopause. She provides a diet plan and recipes in the book (see Resources). There is also a relatively new area of research exploring the relationship between nutrition and mental health. Researchers are demonstrating growing evidence of the impact of nutrition on mood.[8] The British Nutrition Foundation points out that if we eat a well thought-through diet, exercise, maintain a healthy body weight, don't smoke, and limit alcohol consumption, we can reduce the severity of menopausal symptoms and reduce the risk of long-term health problems linked to loss of oestrogen, such as heart disease and osteoporosis (thinning bones).

Sleeping well

Sleep is vital to our general wellbeing, and it can be significantly impacted by menopause. I will discuss this in more detail in Chapter 13, which is dedicated to strategies for managing sleep problems.

Values and acceptance

Know your values

We all have values. These represent the principles that are important to us and how we wish to conduct ourselves. Our values can be influenced by our upbringing as well as experiences later in life; they may change over time. If we have a faith, our values are likely grounded in that. But we often don't stop to reflect on our values and to consider to what extent we are living in alignment with them. If there is a disconnect between what we believe in or hold as important and the way we are acting and living, we create what's called a state of cognitive dissonance. Whether we are consciously aware of this or not, it will cause us to feel uneasy and struggle in some areas in our life, often in ways that we might not be able to explain. So having a clear understanding of what our values are across different aspects of our life, such as health, relationship, work and so on, can help us start to think about how we might put ourselves on track with our values, and hence feel more at peace. During the menopausal transition, we might find ourselves re-evaluating our priorities in life and perhaps even find a new sense of purpose.

To identify your values, ask yourself these questions:

- *What do I care about most in life? What would I sacrifice other things for?*
- *How do I want to be spending my time? Which experiences make me feel fulfilled, peaceful and content?*
- *What qualities do I value most in myself and in others?*
- *How do I want to be remembered as a person?*

Although you may initially think this is slightly morbid, a useful exercise in helping you think about how you want to live your life is actually to imagine your death. Have you ever thought about or tried to write your own obituary? Think about what people might say about you would you want that to be different? If so, what needs to change now? What kind of legacy do you want to leave behind?

Developing meaningful goals

Once we have considered our values, we can then identify goals that will take us towards those values. It is important to clarify the difference between goals and values. Goals are things we aim for in the future – to get, have or achieve – and can be ticked off when we've attained or accomplished them. Values, as described above, are beliefs about what we think is important in life – the principles by which we want to live our lives and interact with other people and the world. Values exist in the present and are ongoing, so they do not have a distinct moment when they have been achieved. For example, getting married would be a goal; being a loving and caring partner would be a value.

To ensure our goals are meaningful to us, they should be aligned with what we hold dear, rather than being driven by external factors/others. In ACT, these are called values-directed goals. Goals developed with our values in mind will help us live a more fulfilling life and can be quite grounding during the turbulent phase of menopause. We might hold the value to have good relationships with our loved ones. But while grappling with all the changes we are going through during this transition, we might lose sight of that a little. So, we can set ourselves a value-directed goal to make space to spend quality time with them, thus strengthening our relationships.

Acceptance and letting go

Practising acceptance has long been recognised as a useful tool for wellbeing in spiritual and religious fields. It leads to improved mental health, personal growth and a general sense of wellness.[9] When we speak of acceptance in a psychological context, we are referring to the process of embracing our thoughts, emotions and other internal experiences without judgement. It involves allowing things to simply be – letting any experience (whether positive, neutral or negative) to exist without actively trying to change, deny or avoid it. For most of us, this process does not come easily but requires conscious effort and needs to be practised like any other skill.

Also, it is not a case of either having acceptance or not having it regarding any specific matter – it can be a matter of degree. If complete acceptance is at one end of the scale, at the other end, there is non-acceptance. The latter may show up in our behaviour as resistance, denial, avoidance, over-control and, suppression, or repression of emotions. This is because we often try to avoid things that we find distressing or painful to experience – whether that is thoughts, memories or feelings. This avoidance may feel like it is helping, as it enables us to avoid what is difficult in the short-term. However, these non-acceptance approaches are not helpful for us in the long-term, because they can trap us into unhelpful patterns of thinking and behaviour.

To accept is to relinquish control; to change what we can and accept what we can't. We also need to be clear that acceptance does not mean we should just give up, or passively resign ourselves to a situation that is unacceptable to us, or let people treat us badly or take advantage of us. For example, if someone is being unkind to us, where possible, we might let them know that their behaviour is not acceptable, or remove ourselves from their company in the future. But we can also acknowledge how we are feeling about this treatment – for example we might be sad or angry – and rather than becoming consumed by these feelings, we can notice, accept, and let them go. So, acceptance goes hand-in-hand with letting go. It opens up the opportunity for moving on, change and personal growth.

As to how you practise acceptance, there are many ways that you can approach it, whether from a spiritual or faith-based understanding, or otherwise. And although it may seem elusive, acceptance is an active process. Russ Harris describes the process of acceptance as the 'interweaving and overlapping phases' of:[10]

- Acknowledging – noticing and acknowledging our experience in a non-judgemental manner
- Allowing – letting it just be, giving it permission to stay
- Accommodating – actively making space for the thoughts and feelings and adapting to them

To explain further:
If you find yourself on quicksand, your instant reaction would be to struggle and fight to get out. But that's exactly what you shouldn't do on quicksand as it will pull you down faster. The best thing is to lie back, spread out your weight, keep still, and really be with the quicksand, then you will float to the surface. That's how it is with your distress too – instead of struggling with it, if you just notice your distressing thoughts and feelings and try to be with them, you'll find that you can overcome them and free yourself from them. (You can watch this as a video if you Google *ACT Quicksand Metaphor.*)[11]

Self-care and connection

Looking out for yourself

As discussed in Chapter 7 on self-compassion, it is important for our mental and emotional wellbeing that we extend some degree of warmth and kindness to ourselves, just as we are able to do towards our loved ones. This should include making time for ourselves to do things that help us relax and bring us joy. This will entail giving ourself priority sometimes over other tasks and responsibilities.

Positive human connections

As humans, we need each other. I discussed in Chapter 7 problems related to isolation. Menopause can be an isolating time. While we are dealing with our symptoms, if can be difficult to maintain existing relationships and/or establish new ones. We might be anxious about getting out to meet people or worry we won't be good company. We might avoid making plans for fear of letting others down if we don't feel up to it when the time comes. However, if we push ourselves to go out anyway and join in with things, it can be a good distraction from our problems for a while. We might also meet others who are going through similar experiences and we may benefit from sharing.

How much human contact you need or want will depend on your personality, as some of us seek company more than others. Just spending time with others can be beneficial. But developing deeper and meaningful connections is even more rewarding. Some people might be lucky to have a good social network they have built up over the years. Others might have fewer connections or have lost contact with people but want to increase their social circle. For many, work might be a natural place to do this. Mothers with young children often have increased opportunities for making new friends. For those outside such groups, it can be hard to know where to start to build up a social network. If you feel that you could do with increasing your social circle, you could look for voluntary roles or local community groups doing activities that you like or might want to try, as they often lead to socialising afterwards, which may lead to building friendships.

One of the best things I did last year was to start my women's 'walk and talk' group. Like a lot of people, I had got into the habit of walking more when the Covid lockdowns started. I knew of the health benefits of walking and recalled hearing that walking also gives relief during heavy menstrual periods, which I have found to be true. My main menopausal symptom at the time though was my joint pain, especially in my knees, and I had just learnt that contrary to what I had previously believed that walking is actually good for that too. Although I don't mind walking alone for the me-time and reflective space, I do also like to share when I come across something interesting. Thinking that others might also like to establish a walking routine, and want company, I started my group. We do our two-hour walk at the start of the week, giving us a good boost for the days ahead. It caters for our physical fitness, emotional and general wellbeing, and social connection, as well as getting us in touch with nature as we walk in the local common, making it a good all-round activity!

Connecting with your spiritual side

I discussed in Chapter 4 how spirituality can help us to cope with challenges in life and how it has been shown to lead to positive outcomes in our health and wellbeing. As you will see from the list below, ways for connecting to your spiritual side may overlap with some of the psychological approaches mentioned already. These have evolved from spiritual practices – and are often used effectively by many, regardless of their faith. Spiritual practices for coping with the stresses of life and developing a more hopeful attitude may include:

- paying attention to your emotions – embracing what it means to be human, warts and all
- being open-hearted (feeling empathy) and serving the community (helping others)
- practicing gratitude – makes you focus on and appreciate the positives in life
- meditation – if you have a faith, this may include prayer

- practising mindfulness – encourages you to focus more on the present rather than dwelling on the past or fretting about the future
- spending time in nature – this is grounding and helps put things in perspective

Key points:

For a balanced life, make this your 5-a-day:

- Eat a balanced diet
- Do at least 20-30min exercise
- Do at least one thing that you find enjoyable or meaningful
- Manage your stress levels – breathe/relax/pray/meditate
- Get a good night's sleep

With new practices, the trick is to aim for 'small and steady' progress, not 'boom and bust'

Your turn:

List your **key learning points** from this chapter

Today I am grateful for:

Reviewing my values and getting a clearer picture of what is important to me

Acceptance techniques – from my faith and ACT

Having taken the initiative to start my 'walk and talk' group and enjoying all the benefits it brings me and the others

List two or three things (big or small) you are **grateful for** right now

9 Problem-Solving Strategies

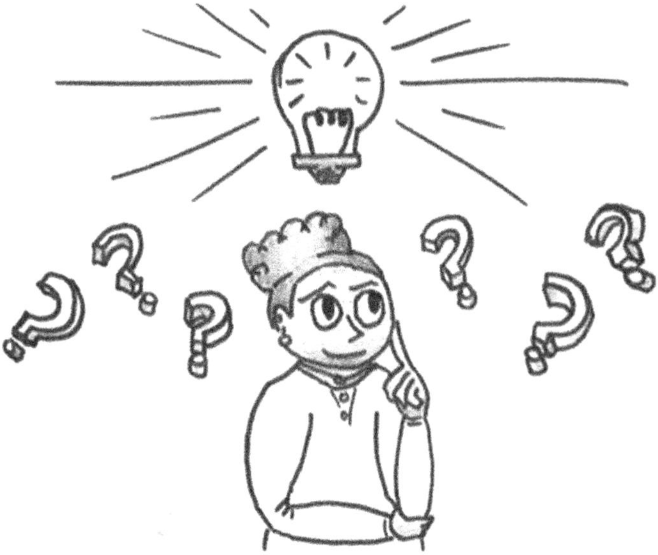

While we may put our best efforts into using strategies like those described in the previous chapter to maintain a healthy and balanced life, they do not make us immune to experiencing some problems along the way. As we know, menopause is constantly throwing new challenges at us. CBT can help us directly tackle these challenges by taking practical approaches to managing problems and learning new coping skills, helping us shift from a sense of overwhelm to that of empowerment.

Within the CBT approach, therapists often talk about helping the client to 'become their own therapist'. The therapist openly shares their thoughts on what they think is happening to the client and their rationale for the choice of techniques they might use and how they work. They collaborate with the client throughout the process; the client can see clearly how it works and can practise this approach even after therapy has ended to continue and maintain their progress. With this concept in mind, I am providing here some generic coping strategies and tools though it is not for therapy in this case. I would describe them more as 'tools for life', in that they may be applied generally for resolving everyday issues. I use them regularly myself and with my clients.

Before we go on to look further at some common menopausal symptoms and how we might approach them from a psychological perspective, I think this is a good point to introduce these problem-solving strategies. Once you understand how they work, you will be able to use them to help you manage different menopausal symptoms. For example, the vicious cycle and coping cycle which were introduced in relation to anxiety in Chapter 6 are further explained here and used in relation to hot flushes in Chapter 10 and brain fog in Chapter 11.

Observing and recording

A practical starting point on the journey of identifying and making changes in your life is to notice and record your thoughts, feelings and behaviours. As I described in Chapter 7, you can use the 'noticing' technique to tune in to your mind and body and observe what is going on for you and how you are responding to difficult situations.

Tracking your menopausal symptoms

As we have seen, the sheer range and fluctuations in menopausal symptoms can make it hard to keep track of them. Putting them down on paper helps to make them feel less overwhelming and gives us a wealth of information to put to use in managing the situation.

One of the first things you might notice are changes in your periods – maybe they are occurring more frequently or less frequently, maybe they are sporadic in their appearance, maybe they are lighter or heavier in flow. By making brief notes on these, you can keep track of the changes occurring in your body. You might also want to record the frequency and intensity of hot flushes and/or night sweats. If you also make notes of what you were doing when they occurred, you might notice that they showed up at certain times of the day under certain circumstances. This will then give you some clues on how you might tackle them.

These records can be helpful for your own understanding, and they can also serve as useful information to share with your doctor to help them understand the history and development of your problems. Being an organised 'lists-person', I've been doing this for years. When I notice myself becoming ill and think I might need to see a doctor, or if I have an upcoming hospital appointment, I'll start making notes about what I observe over time regarding the ailment; I can then see the doctor equipped with my notes. This has been especially helpful in recent years where brain fog can mean I go blank when asked questions in the consulting room. In my experience, healthcare professionals find this helpful as it leads to a more efficient consultation.

Similarly with anxiety and changes in mood, it helps to record how you were feeling in a certain situation, what might have triggered the feeling, what you thought when you were feeling like that and how you reacted or overcame the feeling. This will help you start making links between thoughts, feelings and behaviours, identifying patterns and triggers. Armed with this knowledge, you can start thinking about where and how you might make positive changes. Thinking about the possibility of change can be motivating and empowering. It's like you are in the driving seat and steering things in the direction you want to go.

There is not a specific way of keeping records – you can use diaries, journals, or charts to log your experience of menopausal symptoms. You might want to keep a general log of symptoms as they occur, or if you are particularly troubled by one symptom you might want to focus on that. For example, the frequency and flow of your periods, circumstances when hot flushes occur, or variations in mood. I have given an example in the Menopause Symptoms Experience Log (see Table 9.1), or you can keep notes on your phone. Alternatively, there are numerous mobile apps available, like the Balance App, which has been reviewed and approved by the NHS and other health services around the world.

Defining the problem

The first step in trying to manage any problem is to work out what exactly it is you are trying to deal with. Sometimes you just get the feeling that things 'aren't right' but can't really work out what is actually wrong. You can try and work it out by asking yourself questions like these:

- *What is it that I am finding particularly difficult at the moment?*
- *What is not working like it used to?*
- *What did I used to do and enjoy that I don't do anymore?*
- *What are the good feelings I used to feel that I haven't felt for a while?*

You may find it hard to define this as a single problem or two. It can be helpful to brainstorm with the question, 'What are all the things bothering me right now?' – and write a 'problem list'. Then put this in order of priority from most bothersome or troubling to least. You can then decide which problem you want to start working on first. Don't try to tackle more than one or two problems at the same time, as that will feel overwhelming and make it harder to manage your difficulties.

Often, it can be helpful to start with a simple issue that is fairly easy to manage. When you succeed in resolving one issue, it gives you more confidence to tackle others. For example, you might have been avoiding making an appointment to see the doctor about a perimenopause-related symptom. Ask yourself why you haven't done it yet – is it because you've just been busy with other stuff or is it perhaps because you're worried about what you'll find out. If it's something like not finding the time, remind yourself that it is important to cater to your own needs as much as for others. If it is fear, tell yourself it's preferable to see the doctor and seek

Date/Time/Situation	Symptom Experienced	Duration/Severity	Emotion(s) and Thought Reaction(s)	Behavioural Reaction(s)	Other relevant information
Where was I when I noticed the symptom? What was I doing? What was I wearing? What time of day was it?	*What did I experience? What did I notice in my body?*	*How long did it last? How severe was it? Rate 1-10 (1= least -10 = most)*	*How did I feel when it happened? What went through my mind?*	*What was my immediate reaction? What helped me manage it? Did anything make it worse?*	*Could anything have triggered it? (e.g. activity/food/drink?) Was there anything else significant happening in my life at the time? (e.g. stress at work, argument with friend)*

TABLE 9.1 Menopause Symptoms Experience Log

their advice, thereby potentially allaying your fears and getting the appropriate help sooner rather than later. It might not be as bad as you fear and by seeking help, you are saving yourself more worry. Even if it is bad news, isn't it better to know as early as possible so your doctor can help you to start dealing with it? Once you make that appointment, you are already on the way to dealing with that issue. And that will spur you on to start tackling other things.

Setting achievable goals

Once you know what the problems are, you can go about making plans for how you might deal with them. You will need to think about what kind of outcome you are looking for and set yourself goals. Again, don't try and set more than one or two goals at a time — you want them to be achievable rather than overwhelming. To decide on your goals, you can ask yourself questions like these:

- *Looking at my problem, what needs to change? How do I want things to be different?*
- *What would that look like? How will I feel (physically/mentally/emotionally) different in about 3/6/12 months' time?*
- *What am I willing to do differently to achieve this change?*
- *What practical steps do I need to take?*
- *Realistically, how much time and energy do I have to make this happen?*
- *Do I need to ask for help with some things so I can achieve my aims?*

It's best to start small and step it up gradually. Two areas in which people often struggle are diet and exercise, both of which are important to focus on during menopause. If you are thinking of developing healthier eating habits for example, don't make up an elaborate meal plan and try to follow that straight away. Identify small achievable tweaks to your diet and gradually bring in healthier options over time. Similarly, if you are planning to exercise more, based on the WHO[1] recommendations of 150 minutes of moderate physical activity a week, you would be doing 20 to 30 minutes a day, but this may seem like too much to start with. So, you could start with 5 to 10 minutes of gentle exercises a day, then perhaps build up to doing 30 minutes in three lots of 10 minutes or two lots of 15 minutes and so on, as recommended on numerous NHS Trust websites.

It is good to give yourself timelines for when you want to achieve something, how much effort you need to put in and how often as this helps to keep you focused and motivated. But don't be too strict with yourself. Allow for some flexibility. For example, you might have planned to go for a run three times a week, but you only manage twice during a busy or lazy week. Don't beat yourself up about that, just make more of an effort the following week. When I got myself back into yoga, I started with a 30-day online class, but it took me 36 days as I missed a few here and there – so what! It still set me on the right track with my exercise plan.

Understanding and making links

Drawing out a vicious cycle – Once we have started to notice our thoughts, feelings and behaviour, we may start seeing how they are linked, and the impact that each has on the other. Often, we can get caught up in a negative cycle of thinking. These vicious cycles keep up stuck in a loop and unable to find ways to move forward. All CBT formulations – the way we make sense of what's causing a problem and

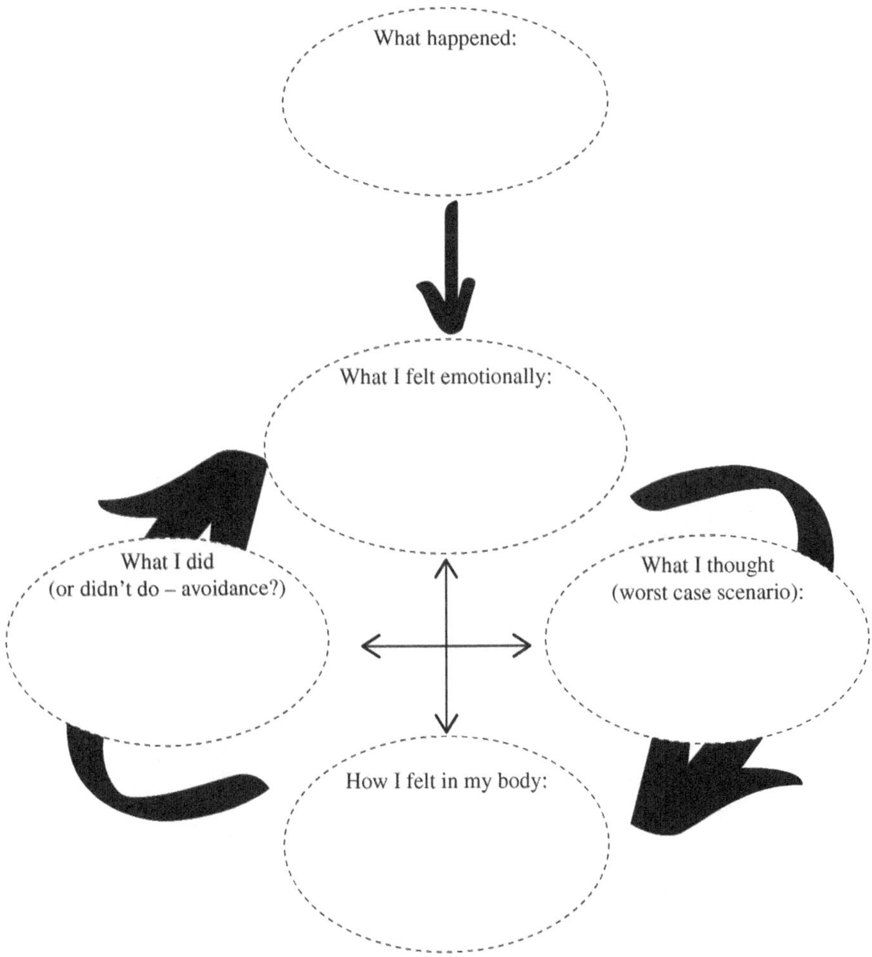

FIGURE 9.1 Vicious Cycle (blank)

keeping it going – are based on the idea of vicious cycles. Once we understand the cycles we are in, we can work towards making changes to break the cycles, and overcome the problem. Any problem can be related to a vicious cycle. Have a look at the examples for anxiety in Chapter 6 and hot flushes in Chapter 10 to see how they work, then fill in the blank one in Figure 9.1 for a situation you might currently be struggling with (there is also another blank one in the Appendix). You can fill in the boxes in any order as they are all interlinked. I usually start with the thing I notice first.

Processing what you find – So, you've been recording for a couple of weeks and seen some unhelpful patterns in your thinking and behaviour. What do you do

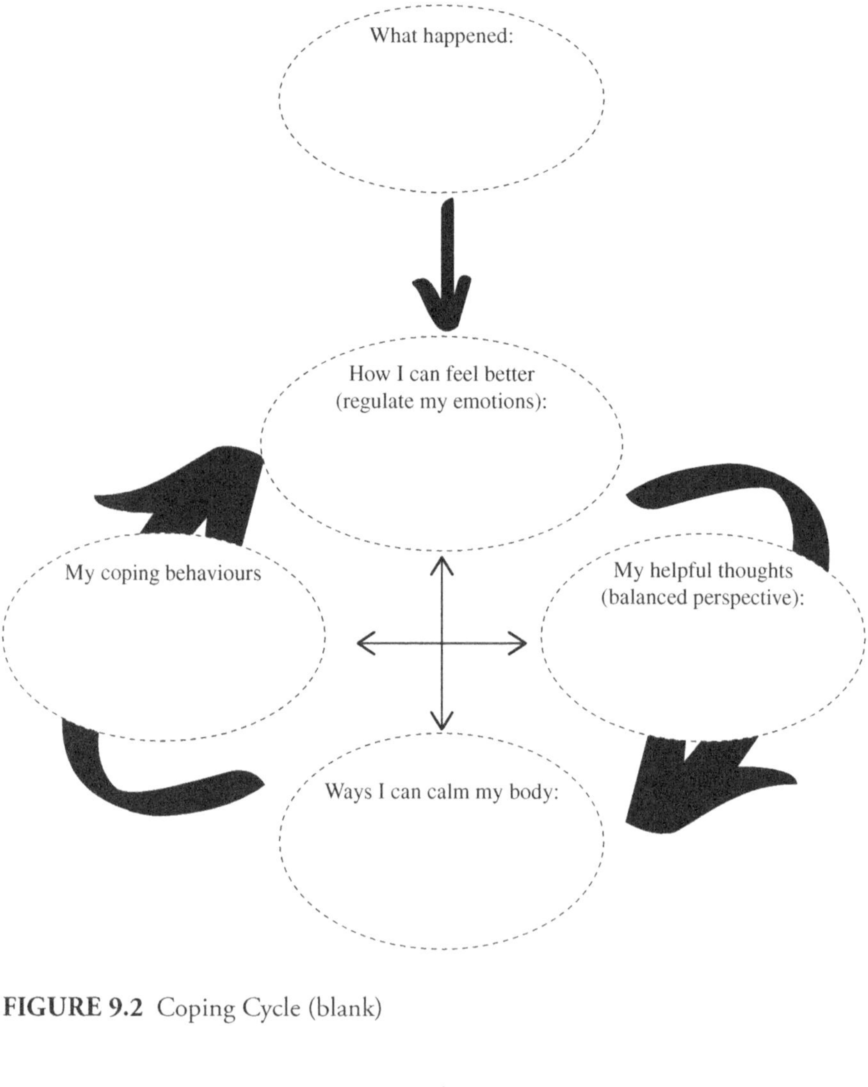

FIGURE 9.2 Coping Cycle (blank)

with this information? First, you might try to 'unhook' yourself from the thoughts (as we discussed in Chapter 6). Then, try to think about other ways you might look at the same situation and develop a more helpful, balanced perspective (also discussed in Chapter 6). After practising the thought challenging techniques, you can re-evaluate your initial thoughts in relation to a given situation. Consider if this re-evaluated thought leads to a different emotion. You can also reconsider your behavioural reaction to it, and then test out a new way of doing things to see how it works out. If it goes well, you can keep practising it until it becomes your more automatic approach, helping you to move forward from the difficulty.

Turning your vicious cycle into a coping cycle – For a given situation, once you have gone through the process of evaluating your thoughts and behaviours and made some changes to break the vicious cycle as described above, you can draw out a coping cycle (see Figure 9.2). This shows how you can develop a more helpful perspective and go on to have a very different experience. See the example in Chapter 6 for anxiety and Chapter 10 for hot flushes. Use the blank one in Figure 9.2 for the situation you completed the vicious cycle for, but of course after having worked through the problem. (Again, there is another blank one in the Appendix)

Charting and maintaining your progress

When you start on any plan of action, it is helpful to keep track of how things are going. For example, if you are implementing changes to your diet or following an exercise plan, you can see if what you are doing is effective. Are your actions taking you towards your intended goal? Charting your progress can motivate you to continue the good work. Alternatively, if you are not seeing signs of progress after a reasonable amount of time, you can go back to the drawing board and consider other ways of getting there. Remember we said to be flexible in your approach. It does not mean you have failed; it just means that approach did not work for you at this time, so try something else that might suit you better. You can develop your own progress chart depending on what it is you are working on and your goals. For example, if you are on an exercise program to build strength, you might log how much time you spend on strength-based exercises and record how much weight you can lift over time (see Chapter 12).

Six-step guide to solving a specific problem

There may be times when you have a problem that needs to be solved rather than a situation to be coped with or dismissed as not worth worrying about. If you take this strategic approach to solving a problem, it can help you feel less overwhelmed as you work towards a solution.

- *Step 1: Identify and define the problem. State the problem as clearly as possible.*
- *Step 2: Generate possible solutions. Give your mind free rein to brainstorm as many solutions as you can think of – don't start worrying about how realistic they are yet...*
- *Step 3: Select and evaluate two or three of your possible solutions, thinking about the pros and cons.*
- *Step 4: Decide what looks like the best solution and make a plan for the steps you need to take.*
- *Step 5: Carry out your plan for the chosen solution.*
- *Step 6: Evaluate the outcome – if the problem is solved, great! If not, think about why it didn't work out, and how you might change certain aspects. If needed, try another of the solutions you came up with.*

Key points:

Tracking your menopausal symptoms is a good way of understanding them

Your records will be valuable data for sharing with healthcare professionals

Charting your progress helps you stay motivated

Today I am grateful for:

My habit of listing and recording which has served me well in **medical consultations**

My realistic diet and exercise goals which I have mostly been able to **stick to, and have seen the health** benefits.

Your turn:

List your **key learning points** from this chapter

List two or three things (big or small) you are **grateful for** right now

10 Vasomotor Symptoms: Hot Flushes and Night Sweats

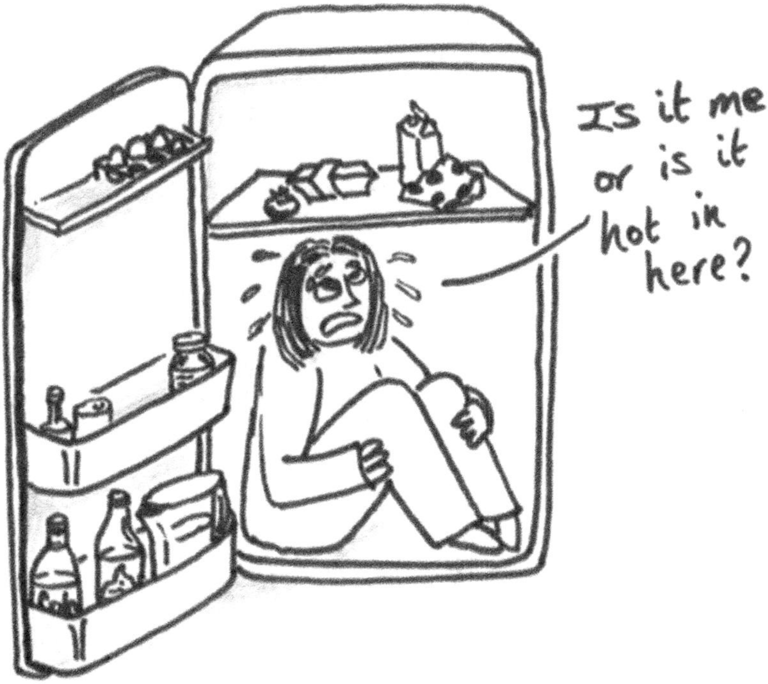

One of the most common features of menopause are temperature regulation problems. These are clinically referred to as vasomotor symptoms because they are reactions in the body which result from changes in blood vessel activity. In common terminology, we are talking about hot flushes (called 'hot flashes' in USA) and night sweats. Sometimes hot flushes can be followed by a cold chill. Aside from the changes in our menstrual cycles, hot flushes are probably the most common symptom during menopause. In fact, it is hot flushes that most frequently comes to mind when people are asked about menopause. A British Menopause Society survey of women in the 45–65 year age-group found that 79% experienced hot flushes. This is probably an under-estimation, as it does not include women who experienced early menopause.[1]

Hot flushes – A hot flush is a sudden feeling of heat radiating through your upper body, typically felt most intensely in the face, neck and chest. You feel very hot, sweaty and flushed, and your skin in those areas may appear red and blotchy. You may notice your heart rate increasing and you may sweat too. Some women also report feeling dizzy and anxious during a hot flush. It comes on very suddenly and can feel very uncomfortable while it lasts. It is their unpredictable nature that makes them particularly hard to manage.

The frequency, intensity and duration of hot flushes vary among women. Some women have them occasionally and are not particularly troubled by them, while others have them more often and can find them quite distressing. They may occur every hour to a couple of times a week, with most women who have them saying they happen daily. They may last anywhere from 30 seconds to 10 minutes, with an average of around 4 minutes.[2] The experiencing of hot flushes can persist for an average of four to seven years, with more than half of women reporting them going on for more than seven years.[3] They can be at their worst towards the end of the perimenopausal phase, then gradually reducing, and possibly continuing to a lesser intensity for up to five years or more post-menopause for approximately 25% of women.[4]

Night sweats – These are hot flushes that happen at night. Their severity can range from your body feeling clammy, to your night clothes being drenched in sweat and even your sheets and mattress feeling soaked. Often, they cause you to wake up from your sleep, and you may need to get out of bed to change out of your night clothes and possibly also change your sheets.

Cold flushes/chills/shivers – This is a less common symptom, but some women experience a sudden extremely cold sensation in their body and find it hard to warm up even with extra layers. Like hot flushes, they can appear out of the blue – for example, when you are in a warm room and suddenly feel a chill and start to shiver. More commonly, you may experience a cold chill immediately after a hot flush or night sweat. This is when the body sweats to cool itself down from the over-heating but the body loses too much heat too quickly. So, at night you may wake up several times from a night sweat when you throw off the covers because you are overheated and sweating, then within minutes, you're pulling the covers back on again because you feel so cold. This can result in poor sleep and subsequent tiredness/low mood/irritability the next day. Cold flushes usually last a few minutes, but can go on for significantly longer.

What causes vasomotor symptoms?

Fluctuating hormones – Scientists are still not entirely sure what causes hot flushes, suggesting they are due to hormonal changes during the menopausal transition.

The part of the brain called the hypothalamus regulates your body temperature. Oestrogen also has a role in modulating your body temperature. It is thought that when oestrogen levels drop, this causes the hypothalamus to become more sensitive to slight changes in body temperature. When the hypothalamus sends a signal that your body is overheated, it triggers a chain of events aimed at cooling you down. This involves the blood vessels near the surface of the skin dilating to increase blood flow to the surface to try to reduce the body heat. If you have fair skin, this may show up as a redness in your face and neck, giving you a flushed look. It may also make you sweat, as the body further attempts to cool itself down.

Night sweats occur at the end of a hot flush when you are sleeping, as you can get overheated under your bed covers and your sweat glands release sweat to cool you down even more. This excessive sweating can leave you with a drenched body and soggy bed clothes.

Cold flushes are even less understood than hot flushes and are assumed to be caused by the same factors – hormone imbalances that cause the hypothalamus to be over-sensitive to temperature changes in the body.

Anxiety – You might ask what came first – the hot flush or the anxiety? Does anxiety cause hot flushes or the other way around? The answer is that it can happen both ways. One longitudinal study (meaning that the participants were followed over a period of time, in this case six years) on the role of anxiety and hormonal changes in menopausal hot flushes found that not only did anxiety precede hot flushes, but women with anxiety were three to five times more likely to have hot flushes.[5] A follow-up to that study (around 10 years later) with 233 of the original 436 participants looked at whether anxiety could be considered a risk factor for menopausal hot flushes. This time the researchers differentiated between affective anxiety (emotional worry) and somatic anxiety (anxiety with physical symptoms). They concluded that while those with affective anxiety were not at greater risk for hot flushes, those with somatic anxiety were much more likely to experience hot flushes throughout their menopausal transition. So, targeting somatic anxiety could help to manage hot flushes.[6]

We also know that hot flushes can *lead* to feelings of anxiety. When a hot flush hits, that sudden sensation of warmth flooding your upper body, increased heart rate and sweating can be incredibly distressing. And being caught off guard because it comes out of the blue can make you anxious. Also, if it occurs in a public place or in a situation where you feel compromised in the presence of others, it can cause embarrassment and worry about the same thing happening again in the future.

Other possible causes – There are a number of other factors thought to give rise to hot flushes, such as: smoking, excessive alcohol, caffeine consumption and spicy foods; prescription medication such as those for breast cancer or osteoporosis or some anti-depressants; and infections or thyroid disease. Also, research has consistently shown women with higher body-mass indexes tend to experience worse hot flushes than thinner women.[7] Some experts say this is because body fat acts as an insulator and prevents heat from escaping, increasing the likelihood of experiencing a hot flush.[8]

You should not automatically assume that your hot flushes are due to menopause if there is a possibility it could be due to other causes. It is best to consult with your doctor who can consider all possibilities.

My meno moments

Climate change you say! Well, let me tell you about heat waves and hot flushes!

- It took a while of asking, 'Is it me or is it hot in here?' and sometimes shouting out at my family, 'Who put the heating on!?' only to touch a radiator and find it was stone cold before I realised it *was* me! On a positive note, during the Autumn 2022 energy crisis, my hot flushes making me turn down the heating made my household pretty energy efficient!
- It wasn't exactly fun when my hot flushes turned up during the summer heatwaves! I recall one such hot July afternoon, working against the clock to get a court report completed having hot flushes for what seemed like every 10 minutes. At the same time, my laptop had a temperamental fan, and it would occasionally overheat and shut down – as if it was having sympathetic hot flushes with me.
- Family summer weddings became a bit of a chore to get dressed up for. I tend to go for the traditional dress of a saree and the paraphernalia (bodice-tight blouse, heels and jewellery) to go with it. For me, dressing up is the best part about attending a wedding. Due of the faff of getting my saree to sit just right, I tend to do my bathroom 'business' before putting it on, then try to avoid needing the bathroom afterwards. I remember getting all dressed up one hot summer's day and then suddenly getting a heavy menstrual flow and a hot flush occurred at the same time – I just wanted to rip everything off and not bother going to the wedding. Talking of ripping everything off, one Saturday afternoon, while bra-shopping in a large department store, I discovered the amazing sense of relief in getting undressed in the fitting room. I might remember that for next time I get a hot flush on a shopping trip – grab a few items off the rack, find the fitting rooms and sit there in my underwear until I've cooled down!
- Then came the night sweats. When I first got these on a January night, I thought I might have Covid. But I did not have other symptoms and tested negative. A few months earlier, when I actually had Covid, I had a fever for two or three days, and though I did sweat, it was nothing like the night

sweats. Again, I had no idea that getting hot and sweaty while sleeping could be related to menopause or hot flushes. I woke up so sweaty I could actually see the drops of perspiration sitting on my neck and chest. My back had sweated through my nightie to my bedsheets. Even my pillow was wet from my head sweating. It was as if I had been in a sauna for far too long. I had to get out of bed, change my night clothes and put a towel under me, as I couldn't change my sheets with my husband fast asleep on the other half of the bed. I had such night sweats nearly every night for a good few weeks. And the disrupted sleep left me exhausted during the day.

- As if hot flushes and night sweats were not horrible enough, the thing I found to be even worse was the discomfort of the night sweats followed by what I called 'the chills'. This was an immediate feeling of cold which felt like a chill right through to my bones. I used to feel this every time I woke from a night sweat. It was like being thrown out of an oven into a freezer. And on many mornings, I would get just the chills as soon as I became conscious on waking up without the night sweats. I would start the day with a chill so severe that I felt frozen stiff and would grit my teeth through it for about a minute or two. And it's not just at night, I also got the occasional chill during the day. And sometimes I got a sort of combo – feeling a hot flush in my neck and chest but a chill in my bones at the same time! I've always been good at multi-tasking!

Coping strategies

Hot flushes cannot be prevented or 'cured', but they do tend to go away eventually. If you only have a few occasional mild hot flushes, you might not need to do anything about them. However, when they are frequent, intense and distressing, you don't have to suffer them – there are treatment options like HRT as well as lots you can do yourself to reduce the frequency and intensity of hot flushes to get some relief from the discomfort they cause. The approach you choose to take will depend on how bothersome they are for you, what approach you feel comfortable with and what sort of behavioural changes you are willing or able to implement. While CBT techniques will not eliminate hot flushes or night sweats, they can give you tools to help deal with the distress you experience and improve your ability to cope.

Identify and reduce or avoid triggers

Understanding how and why hot flushes happen for you will help you be more prepared in managing them. You can track when and where hot flushes occur, what you ate or drank, what you were doing and how you felt just before you experienced a hot flush by keeping simple notes or using the Menopausal Symptoms Experience Log described in Chapter 9. Such records can help you identify if there is a pattern to them – for example, do you get more hot flushes in the evenings or mornings? Are you more prone to them when you are tired, anxious or distressed? Do they come on after eating spicy food or drinking caffeine or alcohol (all known common triggers)? Once you understand what the triggers and patterns are, you can plan how you might avoid or reduce these situations or behaviours with the aim of reducing the intensity and/or frequency of your hot flushes.

Reduce stress and anxiety

As we have seen, research has shown that there is a link between anxiety and hot flushes. We have also seen that somatic anxiety (the physical manifestation of anxiety), in particular, can lead to hot flushes. So, if this is your experience, it would make sense that using techniques for reducing external pressures and anxiety should also help reduce hot flushes. I certainly noticed that to be the case for me. During the summer of 'hot flushes and heatwaves' I described earlier, I had lots going on at work and in my personal life, so I had to take stock and review where I could cut down on some of the pressures. And the thought of getting hot flushes at a 'bad time' made me particularly anxious, which of course only made my hot flushes more likely, so I had to work on managing my anxiety too.

I have taken some of my thoughts and those commonly mentioned by others to demonstrate an example of a vicious cycle of hot flushes in a work situation in Figure 10.1. You can use the blank one in Chapter 9 (or in the Appendix) to draw up your own vicious cycle.

We need to look at our interpretation of the situation, the unhelpful thoughts. If you look at the thoughts recorded in the cycle, you will see that they are quite 'catastrophic'. Using questions such as those mentioned under 'challenging unhelpful thoughts' in Chapter 6, you need to evaluate whether your thoughts are realistic or whether they are just a reflection of your anxiety. For example: Why should I be embarrassed about a natural occurrence like a hot flush; Is there any evidence to suggest that just because I am having a hot flush, people will think I am not capable of doing my job; could they even fire me for such a reason?

You can then do some cognitive restructuring here, that is, to replace your 'catastrophic' thinking with more balanced, helpful thoughts, thus putting things into perspective (see the challenging thoughts section in Chapter 6). Here are a few examples:

- *'I can't cope with these hot flushes!*
  Q: Is that true?
  A: 'Well, I got through the last one. Let's deal with them one at a time.'

- *'These hot flushes are ruining my life!*
  Q: Is that true/helpful?
  A: 'Well, they're not pleasant, but most of them aren't that bad. They do go away. And I've learnt some coping strategies, so they don't have to stop me doing what I want.

When we do this, we will find that our mind and body become calmer, that we become less anxious, which in time will likely also lead to reduced hot flushes in these situations. Figure 10.2 shows what things can look like when these changes are made – I have called it the coping cycle for hot flushes. You can use the blank one in Chapter 9 (or in the Appendix) to draw up your own coping cycle.

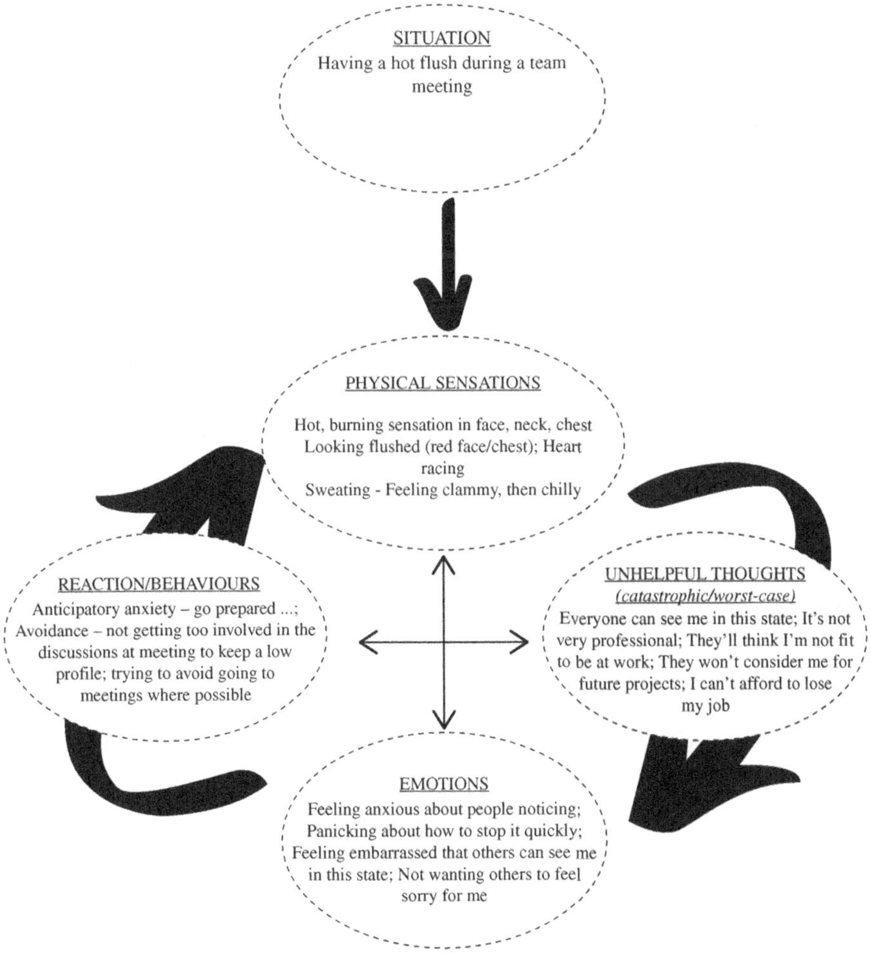

FIGURE 10.1 Vicious Cycle of Hot Flushes

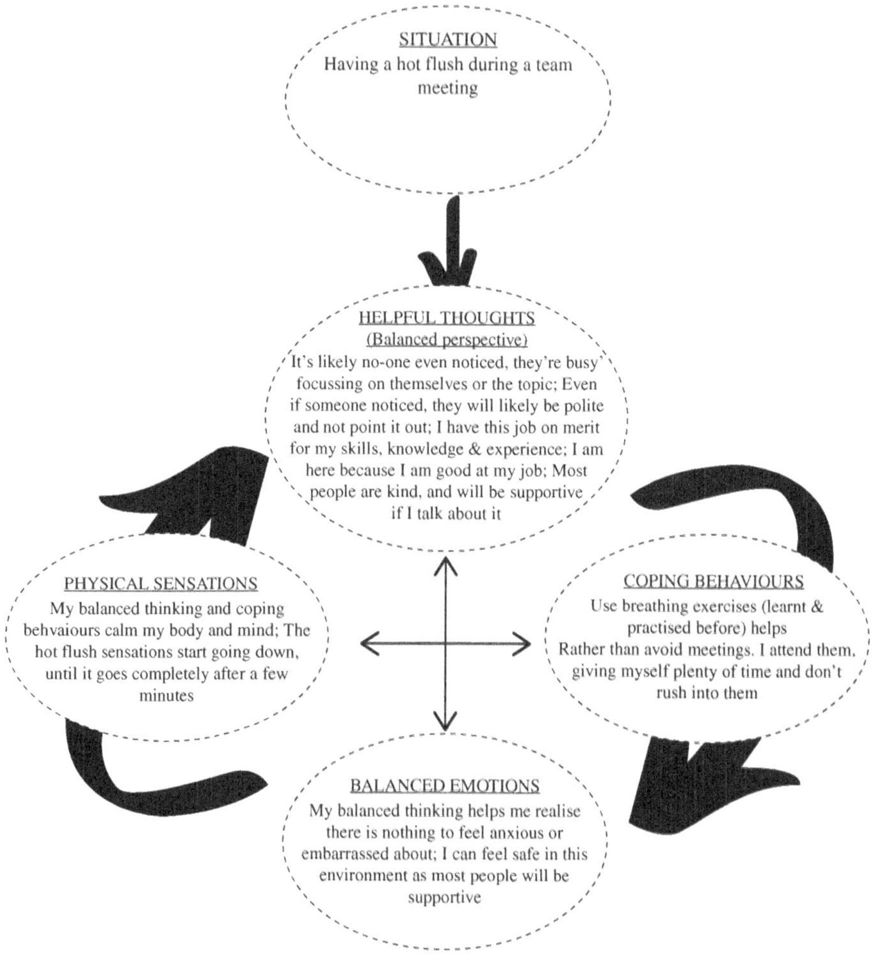

FIGURE 10.2 Coping Cycle of Hot Flushes

Practise paced breathing

Research findings suggest that paced breathing can reduce the intensity of hot flushes, especially if you do them when you first notice the hot flush coming on. Paced breathing is slow, deep, rhythmic breathing which involves purposefully slowing down your breath to focus on the length of the breath and calming your mind and body. As mentioned with anxiety, it is best to practise the technique regularly and make it into a habit rather than just trying to use it when you get a hot flush.[9] When you notice a hot flush coming on, you can use the diaphragmatic breathing exercise described in Chapter 6. Here is

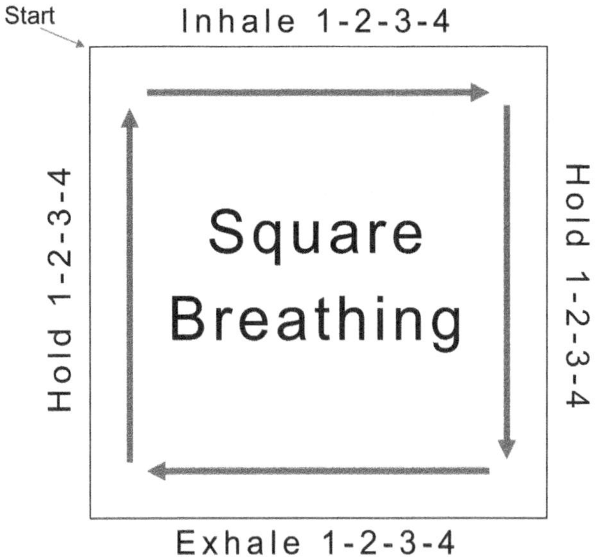

FIGURE 10.3 Square Breathing

another exercise that you can practise called square breathing (also known as box-breathing) (see Figure 10.3):

1. *Sit in a straight-back chair with both feet on the floor, and rest your hands on your abdomen.*
2. *Breathe out slowly, releasing all the air from your lungs.*
3. *Imagine a line drawing of a square and starting at the top left corner, imagine you are moving along the top line as you breathe in through your nose as you slowly count to four in your head.*
4. *Imagine yourself travelling down the line on the right as you hold your breath for a count of four.*
5. *Imagine you travelling left to right along the bottom line while exhaling for another count of four.*
6. *Hold your breath again for a count of four as your breath travels up the final line of the square, back to the starting point.*
7. *Repeat three to four times around the square.*

Guided imagery meditation

Considering the link between stress/anxiety and hot flushes, using meditation and relaxation practices that help lower the stress hormone cortisol[10] can help make you less prone to hot flushes. These tools can be incorporated into your lifestyle for general health and mental wellbeing. I described a relaxation exercise for anxiety management in Chapter 6, which you can also use when you experience a hot flush. Guided imagery techniques have also been shown to help us manage difficult thoughts and feelings and get to a state of relaxation. When I say 'images' in this case, I don't just mean visual depictions of experiences, but also sounds, smells, and other sensory information that run through your mind when you have a thought or feeling. Imagery has the power to influence your emotions and behaviour. Positive images lead to positive emotions and enable you to see yourself doing things differently and more likely to adopt new coping skills to work through difficult emotions or situations.

You can practise guided imagery meditation as a regular relaxation exercise or in times of stress, like when you have a hot flush to calm your body and mind by taking yourself to a place you find soothing and relaxing. You start by doing a breathing exercise like the square-breathing described above, and then you visualise yourself at a scene where you feel at peace and relaxed. It can be a place you have been to or one created purely from your imagination. Examples might include being at the beach, relaxing in a forest or in a field of flowers, or being at a waterfall or mountainside. You can also imagine yourself doing something you love, like dancing, baking or playing the piano. Whatever you choose to visualise, really immerse yourself in the image, using all your senses, so you feel like you are actually there.

Let me take you on one of my favourite walks – in a 'secret garden' within a London common on a spring morning:

- *Choose a quiet time and place. Make yourself comfortable, sitting in a chair or lying down. Close your eyes. Take a few slow, even breaths and focus on just your breath. Breathe in; breathe out. If your attention drifts, gently guide it back – until you feel relaxed.*
- ***SEE:***

  Picture yourself in a secret garden on a spring morning. There is no one else around.

  You are surrounded by the canopy of trees, with leaves of different shades and designs, gently fluttering in a breeze.

  See the beautiful soft colours of the flowers as you walk past them – peach, pink, violet, yellow, and white. Look at the shrubs and grass, soft and fresh with silvery drops of dew sitting on them.

  See the glimpse of the sky through the leaves, clear and blue with one or two soft white fluffy clouds floating by.

  Let yourself sink into the feeling of relaxation.

- ***SMELL:***
  Breathe in and smell the comforting earthiness of the trees and the soil. Smell the fresh 'green-ness' of the shrubs and grass surrounding you.
  Breathe in and smell the fragrance of all the different flowers as you walk past them, collectively letting out a rich perfume.
  Sink a little deeper into relaxation.
- ***LISTEN:***
  Notice the rustling of the leaves and pay attention to the sweet symphony of birdsong.
  Listen to the sound of the water gently flowing over the stones in the nearby stream.
  Feel yourself relaxing even deeper.
- ***FEEL:***
  Feel the spring breeze as it gently sweeps past your face and through your hair. Perhaps the day has not quite warmed up yet so you can feel the breeze on your body too – embrace it. Stay with these feelings and images for as long as you want, taking it all in, and enjoying the experience. Notice how calm and relaxed you feel. Relish the feeling of relaxation as it spreads throughout your body.
- *Notice how distant you feel from any stress or anxiety or distress. Stay here for as long as you like. When you are ready, prepare to leave your tranquil place, and return to the present moment. Slowly count backwards from 10 to zero, then open your eyes, feeling relaxed but alert. Take a few moments to readjust to where you are before moving up.*
- *It may be difficult to visualise an image or control your thoughts when you first begin. If your mind wanders, keep gently guiding yourself back. The more you practice, the easier it will become. Set aside a few minutes every day to help you become more familiar with the practice.*

Grounding

When you are in the midst of a hot flush, it can be so all-encompassing that you feel quite disoriented or detached, like you are removed from that moment and space. I explained how mindfulness helps in coping with stressful situations by keeping you in contact with the present moment. The following A-C-E technique can help you steady yourself and feel more grounded:

- *Acknowledge your thoughts and feelings – gently observe and acknowledge what is 'showing up' within you. For example, you might think, 'This is uncomfortable'; 'I really don't like how I'm sweating so much'.*
- *Come back into and connect with your physical body. For example, wriggling your toes; gently pressing your fingertips together; straightening up your back. The idea is to both be aware of your thoughts and feelings as well as being aware of your body as you move it.*
- *Engage in what you were doing – get a sense of where you are and refocus your attention to what you were doing before the hot flush took over. You could do this in the following ways:*
  - *Look around the room and notice four things you see*
  - *Notice three things you hear*
  - *Notice two things you can smell*
  - *Notice what you can smell/taste/sense in your mouth*
  - *Notice what you are doing*

  It is important to do all three of the ACE steps in order to benefit from this as a grounding technique rather than it becoming a distraction exercise, which would not be as helpful.

(Adapted from Harris, 2019[11])

Holding yourself kindly

As discussed earlier, during hot flushes, we can have unhelpful and/or self-critical thoughts, especially when they occur in the presence of others, because we may be worried about how others perceive us. But we can ask ourselves this: How would I react if my sister or best friend was having a hot flush in front of me? Would I tell her to 'sort herself out'? So, why do we say things like that to ourselves? I described the rationale behind developing self-compassion in Chapter 7. The ACT concept of 'holding yourself kindly' teaches you to show some warmth and compassion to yourself, like giving yourself a hug. Try crossing your arms over your chest so your hands are on your collarbones and your fingertips point towards your shoulders. Rest them there gently for a minute and feel the warmth of your own caress.

Have a go at this exercise I have called the 'soothing hand':

- *So, you've just had a hot flush. Sit yourself down in a comfortable position. Reflect on what you have just experienced. Use the noticing skills described earlier (Chapter 7) to be curious and get a sense of the difficult thoughts and feelings it has brought up for you. Where on your body do you 'feel' the distress of the experience – face, neck, chest, abdomen?*

- *Now, hold up one of your hands (the one you would use to help a child across the road), and turn it palm upwards. Think about times when you might have used this hand in kind and loving ways – for example, to comfort someone who is upset, to check a loved one's forehead for fever or stroking a cat. Now imagine this hand filling up with that same sense of warmth and kindness.*
- *Place this hand gently on the part of your body where you feel the distress. Allow your hand to rest there softly; feel it against your skin or on your clothes, the warmth flowing from your palm into your body. Let the warmth radiate out all over your body, and imagine your body softening and loosening up as it is soothed by your warm, kind hand.*
- *Now, use both of your hands – gently resting one on your chest and the other on your stomach – and hold yourself kindly. You can stay in this position, comforting yourself for as long as you want. (Adapted from Harris, 2019[12])*

Practical solutions

I thought it might also be helpful to give you some tips on practical ways of fending off the very tangible hot flushes. Here are a few suggestions from my experience:

- *Staying hydrated and cool* – During a hot flush, when the sensation of heat escalates, it helps to drink cold water, spray your face with chilled water, or use a cold gel pack. You could also open windows and use fans.
- *Adapting clothes and bedding materials* – Layers of light clothes in natural fabrics like cotton, which is more breathable, are best for adjusting according to changes in your body temperature. I can't tell you how many times I take my layers on and off during my daily 30-minute walks! Likewise, with bedding, cotton sheets and layers of covers rather than a duvet are helpful for adjusting as needed. This reminds me of my pet peeve regarding hotel bedding. Why do they always make the bed with a thick duvet even in the middle of summer? After many a restless night, I learnt to remove the cover from the duvet before going to bed so I can use just the cover if I get too hot. Another bedding tip for night sweats is to place a towel under you so you are prepared to catch the sweat. This makes it easier to replace the towel in the night rather than changing the sheets, which can prove difficult if you have a sleeping partner in the other half of the bed!

- *Turning to technology* – Fabrics incorporating 'moisture-wicking' properties, which are usually used in sportwear, are now being marketed to menopausal women. They are engineered to pull moisture away from the skin to the outer surface of the fabric and into the air, so the fabric dries quickly before it is soaked in sweat, thus easing the discomfort caused by hot flushes and night sweats. I have tried one brand for nightwear which was comfortable and fairly cooling. Sheets and pillows are also available with cooling properties. I have to say that since I started using my 'temperature balancing, smart cool' mattress protector, I have actually not had any heavy soaking-through-sheets night sweats.

Key points

What does a hot flush look like?

Sudden hot or burning feeling spreading the face, neck and chest
A flushed appearance, possibly with red, blotchy skin
Rapid heartbeat
Sweating, mostly on your upper body
A clammy or chilled feeling as the body cools down
Feelings of anxiety or embarrassment

Although hot flushes are unpleasant, there are many ways to manage them

Today I am grateful for:

Having worked out my coping cycle for hot flush situations

My special mattress cover...

Having built a habit of practising yoga as a general wellbeing exercise

Your turn:

List your **key learning points** from this chapter

List two or three things (big or small) you are **grateful for** right now

11 Cognitive Difficulties (Brain Fog)

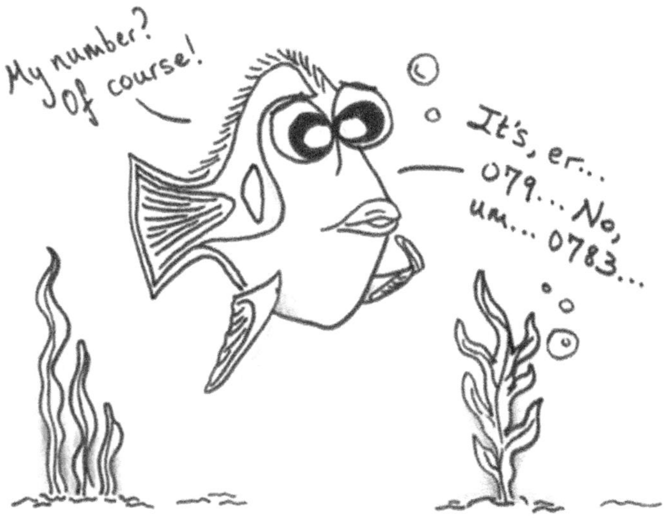
My number? Of course!
It's, er... 079... No, um... 0783...

Problems with cognitive functioning, that is thinking and memory, are a common experience during the menopausal transition, with around 70% of women in the UK reporting a decline in their thinking and memory performance.[1,2] Of course, as with all menopausal symptoms, the extent of the problems experienced will vary between individuals. Some of us may only experience a brief period of occasional forgetfulness, while others become significantly unsettled by our symptoms. The term 'brain fog' is used to encompass the range of cognitive difficulties we might experience, which can include:

- Forgetfulness – needing more reminders than usual or repeating ourselves because we have forgotten what we said
- Concentration problems – finding it hard to focus on a specific task and generally paying attention
- Hazy or foggy memory – feelings of confusion
- Difficulty finding words – having trouble retrieving verbal information, like people's names

- Reduced verbal learning skills
- Mental fatigue – feeling less alert than usual
- Reduced capacity to multi-task

For those who have never experienced brain fog, this is the best way I can think of making it relatable: Imagine you've had a very vivid dream. On immediately waking, you could probably write down or tell someone what you just dreamt. But have a shower and go down to breakfast or go into work, then try to tell someone about your dream. You are likely to find that it feels like it is within your grasp, but you can't quite get at it – you are not able to describe it enough to give someone else a picture of your dream.

Of course, some people generally have better memories that others, and if you are known as someone with not such a great memory, a bit of forgetfulness may be considered normal. With regard to brain fog, we are talking about when you notice that you are more forgetful than usual and are picking up on other difficulties. Although menopause coincides with the time of ageing when we might naturally observe some memory problems, research has shown that ageing alone may not account for the cognitive problems we experience during menopause (see below). Inevitably, by a certain age, we all do the thing where we forget what we came in the room for, or the next level, opening the fridge door and forgetting what we wanted to take out. But with menopausal brain fog, it can become more extreme than that. There were times I didn't even make it to the kitchen, like when I would get up from my chair to go and get something, then have to sit down again as I had instantly forgotten what I was going for. There have been more than a few times that I've started looking around for my phone when I'm actually on it on an online video call.

It also seems that some of our cognitive functions are more affected than others in menopausal brain fog. Verbal memory (the memory for words) seems to be most susceptible, with verbal recall more affected than other types of memory retrieval. This would show up as forgetting an appointment or other planned activity, for example, especially if they were verbally agreed and not written down. There also appears to be a slowing of the brain's processing speed more than loss of executive brain functions. So, we might be more forgetful and be unable to bring to the forefront words that feel like they are just on the tip of the tongue, but we are more likely to retain the capacity to plan and strategise.

Is menopausal brain fog linked to dementia?

Although we would generally associate more serious memory problems with a much older demographic, when we start noticing our menopausal cognitive problems, it is common to start worrying that it might be a sign of something more serious. For me, it started with my family pointing out things like me forgetting I had said or done something, and so repeating myself. Then I started noticing things for myself, such as having trouble finding words and remembering names. Oblivious to being in perimenopause at the time, I suspected I was developing some form of early dementia, because that was the only 'explanation' I could think of. Since then, I have heard so many women, even medically qualified ones, say that they initially thought they were 'losing [their] mind' or developing dementia.

Firstly, we have to remind ourselves that there might be many causes for brain fog. Secondly, there is a difference between the muddled thinking you get with brain fog and the cognitive problems associated with dementia. With respect to the finding that perimenopausal women worry about early onset dementia particularly if they have a family history of dementia, the charity Dementia UK, helpfully point out that when those with early onset dementia (before the age of 65), 'do experience memory and concentration problems, these are not usually early symptoms; changes in vision and spatial awareness, language problems and changes in behaviour are more common in the initial stages'. So, in general, cognitive changes at menopause should not be confused with dementia. Dementia before age 64 years is rare.[3]

As it can be difficult to tell if symptoms are related to menopause, early onset dementia or both, and there are other conditions that can cause dementia-like symptoms, anyone still concerned should seek medical advice for investigation of other potential causes. The same goes for if you your brain fog symptoms persist well into postmenopause. Unless and until we are well informed about these differences, worrying about dementia can cause anxiety, which in turn can have an impact on our cognition, such as making it harder to focus or concentrate on things, creating a vicious cycle.

There is reassurance from research that the level of decline in our cognitive abilities during menopause is minimal and that our abilities remain within normal range. One research of 400 women studied over several years, found that about one-third experienced a clinically significant decline in memory following menopause, but that even in those women, the level of decline was not indicative of dementia.[4] Another piece of reassuring news is the research suggesting that when we reach the postmenopausal stage, memory difficulties (especially in verbal memory skills) may resolve for many of us.[5] So, the symptoms we experience during perimenopause will not necessarily follow us into the postmenopausal years. It's good to know that the fog is likely to clear. So, I guess I'll hold off my application to go on as a contestant on 'Pointless' (TV quiz show) until then – though I must say I am pretty good at it even with the brain fog, well from my armchair anyway!

What causes brain fog?

As with other menopausal symptoms, brain fog may be caused by a number of factors:

Fluctuation in oestrogen levels – Oestrogen encourages blood flow to the brain which is loaded with oestrogen receptors, particularly in the memory storage and processing areas. Oestrogen stimulates the brain, keeps the production of new cells going and maintains the efficiency of existing brain cells. So, oestrogen plays a role in brain processes such as language skills, memory and attention skills, and when the level of oestrogen in our body fluctuates, it affects our brain's capacity to function.[5]

Reduction in other hormone levels – The female body needs the hormone testosterone, especially for the brain. Testosterone helps supply the brain with blood, which is essential for preventing memory loss. It strengthens the nerves in our brain and enables mental clarity and sharpness. So, insufficient testosterone levels can have an impact on brain functioning. Decline in follicle-stimulating hormone (FSH) has also been linked to memory problems.[6]

Reduction in blood sugar levels – The hormone changes that occur in the body during perimenopause can drain it of energy, which means a reduction in blood sugar levels. The brain needs glucose to function and as it uses a lot of energy, having less glucose in the body means there is less available for the brain to function at its best. Oestrogen improves memory functions, partly by promoting increased supply of glucose – so as oestrogen declines, the processing time required to store or access memory increases.

Lack of sleep/poor quality of sleep – When we are in deep sleep (the rapid eye movement, or REM, stage), our brain processes all the information from the day and stores our memories. So, if we don't sleep well and get enough deep sleep, this important stage of cognitive activity will be interrupted. Hence, when we are sleep-deprived, we are more prone to experiencing memory loss. As we discussed in Chapter 10, the disruption caused by hot flushes and night sweats can lead to poor quality sleep, and in turn have an impact on our mental acuity during the day.

Stress, anxiety and depression – The experience of brain fog itself can be quite anxiety-provoking and may lead to worry, which can make it harder to focus on things. Anxiety causes simple tasks to appear more difficult. Menopause often coincides with a number of potential life stressors. Stress, whether short term (acute) or longer-term (chronic), can contribute to attention issues and memory loss.[7] This is because, the stress hormone cortisol is known to suppress learning and memory, particularly verbal memory, which is most affected in menopausal brain fog. Stress and anxiety take up more energy in the brain, causing other cognitive functions to suffer. Depression has also been significantly correlated with deficits in:

- Processing speed the fluency with which the brain receives, understands and responds to information
- Verbal memory – the memory for words and association between words
- Working memory – the short-term memory that holds information temporarily while we carry out cognitive tasks like working out a maths problem.[8]

My meno moments

My brain fog experiences have, at times, been particularly bothersome and extremely frustrating, making it one of the most troubling aspects of living through menopause. Let me tell you about my very foggy summer of 2022. From around June to September, I just kept having one cognitive mishap after another. And I was not particularly stressed at the time so I might attribute my memory and concentration problems to being over-burdened. If I hadn't been making journaling notes for this book, I think that period would be a complete blank in my memory, like when people talk about their drunken student years, except that I hadn't even had a drink! You'll be impressed by the variety of ways my brain could get muddled!

- A lot of things I noticed related to the gadgets we all use these days; phones and computers. By the time I'd squiggled my passcode across the screen with my forefinger to unlock my phone I'd forgotten what I was about to do on my phone – was it a text, or WhatsApp message or email? who to? Or, I would click on the Google icon and immediately forget what I was going to look up! I remember re-setting my password for a shopping account where you create a password and type it in twice – I did that, but then, within about 30 seconds, I couldn't remember it to type it again to log in!
- This one really bothered me at the time. I had to call a furniture shop about my sofa delivery and they asked for my number to call me back. I said, 'Yes, of course, it's *07868 599* ... erm …' (I suddenly went blank) '... 078. Erm, no that doesn't sound right … Sorry about this I don't know why I've just gone blank ... Let me see if I can find my number ... I have two phones so must be getting mixed up'. I fumbled around looking for something with my number on it – which didn't seem that easy – and eventually was able to give him my number. I felt glad that he was patient enough to wait for it, but also very annoyed with myself, and saying out loud after the call,

'F***ing hell! I'm going to forget my own bloody name soon!' It made me think of Dory, the fish with amnesia, in the film 'Finding Nemo' (2003) who needs to carry a tag with her name and address on it.

- I was on holiday on a Greek island and spotted an interesting tree that I hadn't expected to find there. I could not name the fruit growing on that tree – it was on the tip of my tongue, and even the Bengali word for it 'tatul', which I would rarely have used came to me first, but despite knowing that, I still couldn't retrieve the English word for it. It bugged me for three days before I finally remembered the word 'tamarind'.
- This next one actually shook me for a few hours: It was a beautiful sunny day and I was driving myself and a friend to a park familiar to me (so I wasn't using the SatNav) thinking about when to turn-off the road, when my mind went absolutely blank. My friend named the park but I couldn't think where I was going at all. I became flustered, not so much because we might take the wrong turn-off, but because I felt so blank. I felt like my brain had just emptied itself out like a skip that's just offloaded building rubble. My anxiety only lasted for about a minute before I was able to recoup myself by taking a couple of deep breaths, and recalled the destination. But it did make me concerned about possible future occurrences like that.
- That same day in the evening, I had been having tea and chatting with my friend at home and after she left, I heard water rushing in the bathroom upstairs. I found I had left the hot water tap running – for three hours! In the middle of an energy bill crisis and hosepipe ban!
- On a cosy night in with my husband, we decided to watch a film. I suggested 'The Wife' (2017) saying I've read the reviews and it sounds good. We started watching it, and I immediately thought it looked a bit familiar but ignored the thought and continued watching. As the film progressed, I couldn't help thinking I knew this story, but at the same time I couldn't really remember what happened next, so I spent a lot of time watching it feeling quite baffled. I thought, 'either this is a very predictable story-line or I must have seen it before?' It wasn't until I got almost to the end of the film that I realised that I had indeed seen it before, and actually only about six months earlier!

Coping strategies

Fortunately, there are lots of practical ways we can manage the challenges of cognitive difficulties and their potential impact on our psychological and emotional wellbeing.

Use memory aids

When short-term memory is affected by brain fog, using memory aids can be effective in helping to retain information.

Notes to self – For the past few years, keeping notes in the memo function of my phone has been my saving grace. In addition to having numerous 'to-do' lists, I have many pages of notes – all the things I have to write down 'before I forget'. Making notes about things like where my important documents are kept, ideas for projects, people to call back and so on. I feel I've become like Leonard Shelby (played by Guy Pearce) in the film 'Memento' (2000). He is trying to work out who killed his wife but is suffering from amnesia. So, he comes up with methods to help him remember – like notes to himself placed in his pockets, photographs and tattoos on his body and a system of colour-coded files to help him keep track of his investigations.

Photographic 'evidence' – As we all have the wonderful tool of a camera on our mobile phones, we can use this to take pictures of things we need to remember, such as the spot in the enormous car park where we parked the car. I also love the screenshot feature on my phone to capture essential information – such as tickets to an event – so I can access them quickly when I need to show them rather than having to search for it in an email.

Setting alarms – I use the alarm feature on my phone to remind myself to do things. Though I often have to write a note of what that action is, otherwise when the alarm goes off, I may struggle to remember what it was for. I have found putting entries of it in my phone diary, giving it a name and setting a reminder useful for more important things.

Make meaningful associations – This can be a useful strategy for recalling information. For example, when being introduced to someone new, listen attentively, immediately repeat the name in your head, and try to make the name 'meaningful' by linking to something that's memorable for you – you might connect their name to a celebrity or someone you know with the same name; or you might make a point of noticing a particular physical feature of the person and 'attaching' it mentally to their name. Last year, I met a woman called Siobhan and the first person I thought of was Siobhan from 'Bananarama' (an all-female pop group from the 1980s). I struggled to remember the surname. I ended up telling her this, and she told me it was Fahy, and that's who her father had named her after as he had a crush on her. We had a nice chat about 'Bananarama', and now whenever I see her or need to mention her, I easily remember her name.

Exercising the brain

The brain is a muscle and just like other muscles in the body, it needs to be kept active. Mental activity will help the mind to stay healthy and working to its best capacity. There are lots of helpful mental exercises we can do to stimulate our memory and strengthen our cognitive abilities, such as reading, doing crosswords, practice word games, doing puzzles, or other activities that require us to think and concentrate. We have a lot of these at out fingertips on our phones, so can easily practice for a few minutes here and there.

Relax – slow down – share burdens

In Chapter 6, I described how practicing a deeper, more paced way of breathing is a helpful anxiety management technique. This calms down our body and mind, so will not only reduce anxiety in general but also the anxiety that comes from experiencing brain fog. When we are stressed with too much to do with too little time or weighed down by the burden of responsibility, it can be hard for our brain to keep up and function optimally. For example, when we are rushing around, we can become flustered, and the more we become flustered, the more likely we are to forget things and the more prone we are to tripping up and making mistakes (another vicious cycle). So, finding healthy ways to manage stress will help in reducing the impact it can have on our memory. The overall idea is to reduce the burdens of responsibility where possible and slowing down.

One way to slow things down is to get organised and do tasks in a strategic and routine manner, hence reducing the strain, feeling more relaxed and less likely to be forgetful. We then find that our brain functions better and we feel better overall. Here are a few simple reminders for reducing stress in your everyday life and lessening the burden on your mind:

- Stop rushing around so much – remind yourself of what the priorities are so you don't get into a mindset that 'everything needs to be done now'. You will achieve more by doing things at a steady pace.
- Ask yourself if you have more to do than time allows – can some tasks be shared or delegated?
- Relax your posture – when you notice yourself tensing up, drop your shoulders and loosen your body with movement.
- Take short breaks – get up, stretch your body, go for a walk.
- Give yourself little things to look forward to – like a call to catch up with a friend.

Re-frame those niggling unhelpful thoughts

Although we may be informed that there are differences between dementia and brain fog, when we experience cloudy thinking, forgetfulness and cognitive mistakes, sometimes we can still get a niggly thought of 'but what if …?' and can set ourselves off towards thinking of all the worst case scenarios. Or even if we are reassured it is not dementia, we can still have 'what if' thoughts about how our brain fog might lead to negative outcomes like messing up at work and maybe even losing our jobs. I discussed in Chapter 6 techniques for becoming aware of our unhelpful thought patterns and challenging or relating to them differently in order to break the vicious cycle or 'unhook' us from them. You can use those techniques here, and perhaps complete a vicious cycle diagram followed by a coping cycle one (use the blank ones in Chapter 9 and in the Appendix). Here are some examples of how 'what if'/ catastrophic thoughts can be positively reframed to help you manage if you become anxious or self-critical during your experience of brain fog:

UNHELPFUL THOUGHTS	HELPFUL THOUGHTS
I'm always forgetting things – what if it is dementia?	I've spoken with my doctor and they ruled out dementia. I am thankful it is not dementia. Brain fog does pass over time.
My head is so fuzzy today, I'm going to mess up my presentation and embarrass myself.	I have prepared and I know what I'm talking about. If I make a mistake, I'll just correct it straight away. It might not even be noticed, but if it is, I'll admit it, apologise, and move on. Mistakes can happen to anyone!
I'm going to meet so many important people at tonight's event; what if I forget their names?	I can manage my anxiety using the strategies I have learnt, so I can be in the moment and pay attention. I know some techniques for remembering names, so I'll be OK. If I do forget, I'll avoid saying their name and someone else will come along and say it.

Sharing with family and friends

It helps to talk to others about what you are going through. If you share with women of similar age, you might find that they are going through or have been through similar experiences which they are happy to share too. It will lighten the load for you and also improve your sense of connection. During my foggy summer, I was on a day out with a friend and told her how I was struggling with brain fog and that this was making it challenging to write a book. She spoke about her own difficulties with brain fog. We had an endearing afternoon helping each other out with words we couldn't find. For example, we were talking about plants and I expressed my frustration at never being able to remember the name of the 'tall feathery plants at the back of my garden nicely hiding the shed, starting with "m" I think ...' After we went through numerous plant names, I felt so excited to finally remember 'bamboo'. Then, she mentioned her journalist partner had gone to, 'now where was it ... the country who's capital is Adis Abbaba'. 'Oh oh, Ethiopia!', I said excitedly. It was a good bonding experience.

It is what it is ...

I think sometimes we can struggle with things because we think they 'should' not be so. We have expectations of how life should go and when things don't match up to that we can feel frustrated, blame ourselves, blame others. But if we can get ourselves to a place of 'acceptance' that it just is the way it is, we may not try so hard to make it not so and let go of the control we try to harness. With each brain fog moment, we can acknowledge that it has happened (notice it, observe the moment with no judgement); allow it to be (we don't have to jump at trying to make the experience 'disappear'); and accommodate it (we can sit with it, maybe even laugh it off) and carry on with whatever we were doing. Acceptance and letting go gives us a sense of relief.

Also, if we learn to be more compassionate with ourselves, as we are with our loved ones, life will be a lot easier. The ACT definition of compassion is to 'acknowledge pain and respond with kindness'. Pain refers to not just physical pain and suffering, but basically anything that goes wrong for us or causes distress. So what if I made a mistake? Or was a bit delayed in finding a word ... It's not such a big deal. I don't have to keep apologising for it ... This will help us to relax a little more in those moments, which in turn is likely to lead to fewer brain fog moments. Now I'm not saying this is easy; it does take a lot of practice. Also, it is a lot easier when you are willing to open up and share with others what you are going through. I recently had another brain fog moment of not being able to provide personal details requested of me in a shop. This time, instead of getting angry with myself about it, I made light of the situation about being menopausal. This resulted in an empathic conversation with the woman I was speaking to about our shared experiences, and even her male colleague joined in talking about the experiences of women in his life.

As you can see from my examples, brain fog can present in so many ways and under all sorts of circumstances. As I noticed these incidences more and more, I started thinking maybe I was better off when I was oblivious to what was going on rather than being aware and spotting it and becoming increasingly frustrated and upset by it. I have had to work hard on myself to accept that things may be like this for a while now so life will be easier if I am more compassionate with myself instead of focusing on how I failed or what I have lost. (See Chapter 7 on self-compassion and Chapter 8 on acceptance.) I believe my developing spirituality over recent years has helped me with this.

Celebrate little successes

Notice and be grateful for when things go well. I make a note in diary when I find words like 'inhibition' and 'serendipity' with little or no struggle, as words like these seem to have become harder to retrieve in the midst of my brain fog. It makes me feel more hopeful. (See how to develop and practice gratitude in Chapter 7.)

Optimising health

Our cognitive abilities are impacted by our physical health. For example, the quality of sleep we are getting, stress and anxiety levels and so on. To maintain and improve brain functioning, we need to look after our health. The best way to do this is to build some structure in our day and establish good routines in our activities of daily functioning (see Chapter 8). Also, when we do physical exercise, it's not just our body we're working on – it improves our mind too. Researchers believe physical activity promotes the release of protein in the brain, which helps in the repair of existing brain cells and the growth of new ones and so maintaining learning and memory functions.[9] One small study found that higher levels of physical activity and cardiorespiratory fitness (aerobic activities like walking, running and cycling) were associated with better cognitive function in postmenopausal women with breast cancer.[10] More clinical trials are needed to look into the impact of physical activity on cognitive function and the mechanisms underlying the benefits for cognitive function in menopausal women.

Improving sleep

As we have said, the poor, disrupted sleep which is common during menopause, can make it hard to focus or learn and retain new information. So, trying to improve the quality of our sleep can help protect the brain against loss of cognitive function. I have always been a bad sleeper and often surprised myself how I managed to get through some days on very little sleep. But when all my perimenopausal problems came to a head, I finally decided that I needed to sort out my sleep and had to accept that bedtime routines are not just for children or for boring people! We need to get sufficient sleep, regular sleep and good quality sleep. To promote deep and restful sleep, we need a sleep routine, as I will discuss in Chapter 13.

Trying to avoid hot flushes

There is some research evidence to suggest that women who experience moderate to severe degree of vasomotor symptoms tend to have more memory problems, especially in their verbal memory.[5] This indicates that if we can avoid hot flushes or reduce their severity, we might also experience less brain fog. (See Chapter 10 for ways to manage hot flushes.)

Key points

There is a difference between menopausal brain fog and dementia

Like the body, the brain needs to be kept healthy and active

Memory function tends to improve again in post-menopause

Today I am grateful for:

Realising that I don't have early onset dementia

Having friends to share, and laugh about, brain fog moments with

My phone – for all the ways it serves as my memory right now

Your turn:

List your **key learning points** from this chapter

List two or three things (big or small) you are **grateful for** right now

12 Weight Gain and Joint Pain

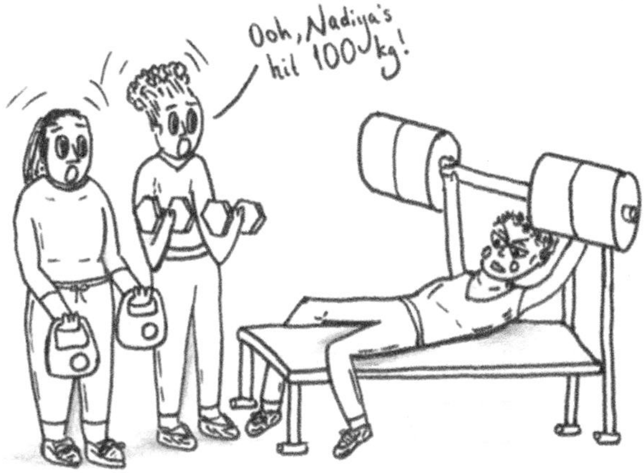

Menopause used to be colloquially referred to as 'the change', presumably alluding to 'the change of life' for a woman in terms of her reproductive capacity. And change, on so many levels, is exactly what is happening, whether it's in our menstrual cycle, our physical appearance or the way our mind and body now react to things.

The list of symptoms in Chapter 1 included numerous physical symptoms and bodily changes that can occur as a part of the menopausal transition. I have experienced a number of these myself, such as thinning hair, dry itchy skin and restless legs. Although I assume there is a link to perimenopause due to hormonal changes at this stage of my life, I cannot be sure some of them are not just part of the ageing process. There are many suggestions for how to manage the physical symptoms, and I would advise you to do your own research and seek advice from an appropriately qualified practitioner.

Two of the changes that I do believe are mainly linked to my perimenopause transition are weight gain and joint pain. So, I have selected these to focus on. That is not to dismiss, all the other physical symptoms that can cause havoc during menopause. It's just that with these, I feel I have something to offer in terms of coping strategies. And these symptoms may often go hand in hand, so the way to manage them can also be a joint effort.

Weight gain and change in body shape

As we get older, we will notice that we struggle to keep to our usual weight – we tend to put it on faster and find it harder to lose. Not all women put on weight in menopause – some might actually lose weight or need to gain some. More commonly though, around half of us start putting on weight during perimenopause and continue into postmenopause. Research indicates that on average women gain approximately 1.5 kg per year during their perimenopause, ending up with an average weight gain of 10 kg by the time they reach menopause.[1,2] And many women, like me, say they have reached their heaviest weight during perimenopause. Even if we manage to keep our weight down and do not gain too much, we may notice a difference in our body shape. This is because the way fat is distributed in our body changes with hormonal fluctuations, and we put the weight on more around our abdomen and upper body.

What causes weight gain?

The weight we might gain during our menopausal years may be due to a number of factors:

Ageing – Menopause coincides with ageing, and as we get older, our muscle mass typically goes down while fat increases. The loss in muscle mass slows down our metabolism and causes weight gain. So, unless we make changes to our diet and exercise more, we are likely to gain weight. Unfortunately, we also tend to become less active as we get older.

Oestrogen and fat distribution – The reduced levels of oestrogen in our body during menopause can cause fat to be stored around our abdomen rather than on our hips and thighs, hence the increased waistline. When we are postmenopausal, this store of belly fat may account for 15 to 20% of our total body weight, compared to 5 to 8% when we are premenopausal.

Menopausal symptoms – Some menopausal symptoms, such as low mood and poor sleep, can also contribute to weight gain. Low mood can make it harder for us to be motivated to exercise and eat more healthily. Insufficient sleep can make us feel too tired to engage in activities and can disrupt the hormones which inform us when we are hungry or full, so we can consume extra calories by snacking more.

General stresses of life – There is often a lot going on for us around this time in our life. These pressures can make us prioritise other things, lose focus on looking after our health or just feel too overwhelmed to find the time even when we are aware of what is needed.

My meno moments

- For the two years of Covid lockdowns, being perimenopausal and working from home, I had put on 'work-smart' tops and not needed to dress my lower half in 'proper clothes', wearing pyjama bottoms and joggers instead. Then when the world started to open up and I needed to go out more, I found most of my skirts and trousers no longer fit. I had reached the heaviest weight I had ever been. Every time I failed to squeeze into an outfit before going out, it would lead to me feeling low in mood and veering between saying, 'F*** it, I'll live in leggings for the rest of my life' and motivating myself into a burst of activity. I refused to buy larger clothes – I decided I had to get the weight off.
- As for my body shape, I recently got a reminder popping up on Facebook of a post I had entitled 'The Tale of the Disappearing Waistline' – I had visited the house of D.H. Lawrence in Eastwood, Nottingham, in 1992 and again 25 years later in 2017, compared photos of myself during those visits, and noticed the stark contrast. But then, I had to remind myself that in the first photo I was 23, when I had a well-defined waistline, and in the second I was 48, having had two children. My figure has gone from being roughly an hourglass (though interestingly, I never thought of my body in that way at the time) to a beer-glass, and I'm currently trying to stop myself turning into a jam-jar. Does it really matter? Well, the shape doesn't matter as long as I am confident in it – looking back it seems I wasn't that confident in my body as an hourglass anyway. The main thing is to be fit and within a healthy weight, and you can be that with any shape. My priority right now is to look after my joints. And I suppose I'll know I have reached acceptance of my new body shape when I clear out of my wardrobe the outfits that no longer fit but I'm still hoping to get back into one day. Then there are those aspirational items – you know, the outfits you fall in love with in the sales and they're a little too tight but you buy them anyway because you plan to fit into them comfortably one day. I seem to even have a pair of shoes in that category at the bottom of my wardrobe – maybe I thought my feet would shrink as I got older and then they'll fit perfectly!

Coping strategies

As with the menopausal journey, we will all be at our own personal stage with regard to our weight. And sometimes it's not a simple case of saying 'just lose some weight', as there may be many reasons why we have put on extra pounds over the years, in addition to the usual ageing and menopausal factors. So, it is really about each of us looking at where we are, and how our weight might be playing a part in our health problems. Then doing what we can to be as fit and healthy as possible.

Good nutrition and weight management

Weight management is not just about going on a diet and losing weight. We need to make sure we eat well, as there are certain nutrients that are more beneficial for us during the menopausal transition and postmenopause. If you decide you do need to lose weight, it's best to avoid restrictive diets which promise fast weight loss in favour of a well-balanced calorie-reducing diet. Once we are in our 50s, we need around 200 fewer calories a day than we did in our 30s and 40s just to stay at our current weight. To lose weight, we may need to reduce calories a little further, but we should do this by paying attention to the nutritional value of what we are eating. Also, any diet should be combined with increased exercise. That is the best way to reduce the waistline and body fat that tends to accumulate during menopause. Of course, you should consult with your GP before starting a significant new diet.

Limit alcohol and sweet drinks

Alcoholic beverages add extra calories. And there are a lot of extra calories in sugar-sweetened beverages, such as soft drinks, juices, energy drinks, flavoured waters and sweetened coffee and tea.

Muscle-building exercise

We gradually lose muscle mass as we get older. And as muscle burns calories, losing muscle means our basal metabolic rate drops – this is the amount of energy or number of calories that your body needs to carry out its basic function. That's why it is harder to lose weight at this age and even to keep at our usual weight if we don't reduce our calories a little. So, during menopause, in addition to general physical activity for wellbeing, we should try to focus on doing regular, consistent, weight resistance exercise as that is the way to build muscle, which will then help us burn calories better and make it easier to manage our weight. Again, do consult with your GP before embarking on a new exercise or fitness regime.

Overcoming psychological factors

We often make good intentions to eat healthier, but can still find it very challenging. There are many factors which can influence our attitude towards food and our eating behaviours – social, cultural, economic status, etc. – and one of the main ones is psychological. Although some people eat less when they experience strong emotions, many people use eating as a coping mechanism to deal with feelings such as stress, boredom, anger, sadness and loneliness. This kind of emotional eating – more commonly called 'comfort eating' – is a form of avoidance. It may suppress or soothe negative emotions in the short term but, because you are not dealing with the underlying issues, it is not a good solution longer term. It often leads to feelings of regret and guilt and may even increase the feelings you were trying to avoid. It can also lead to additional problems, such as poor self-image/low self-esteem as you gain weight or health problems related to the weight gain.

With emotional eating, your emotions can become so tied to your eating habits that you automatically reach for a treat or quickly eat whatever is convenient without thinking about it or actually enjoying it. Habits that have built up over years can be hard to break. It is worth trying to explore the psychological issues that might be holding you back so you can implement changes to help you move forward, as I will go on to discuss. Sometimes the weight issues may be linked to deeper emotional issues that you may need the help of a counsellor or therapist to explore further and address appropriately (see the Further Support and Resources section).

As usual, CBT takes a two-pronged approach:

Cognitive: identifying self-defeating thinking patterns that contribute to weight management problems.

Behavioural: identifying eating patterns and changing to healthier eating behaviours.

You can use the 'noticing' technique (see Chapter 7) to tap into your emotions and thoughts and the challenging and cognitive restructuring approach to re-evaluate your perspective (see Chapter 6). You can draw your experience out as vicious and coping cycles, as you've seen elsewhere in the book. Then you will have a more balanced, helpful way of thinking and responding. For example:

Self-defeating thought	***Positively re-framed statement***
It's too hard. I can't do it.	I know I am overeating, but I can look into *how* I can change this.
If I don't reach my target weight, I have failed.	I need to identify what triggers my overeating, then plan a way to manage this.
Now that I've lost weight, I can go back to eating anything I like.	I can't undo the hard work I've put in. My craving should pass if I delay eating by doing something else for a while.

Keep a 'food and feelings' diary

I discussed recording and observation in Chapter 9. A simple food diary is often a starting point for watching what you eat in terms of having regular and nutritionally balanced meals. However, if you also incorporate tracking your food intake in relation to situations, thoughts and feelings, it can help you work out what is helpful and unhelpful in your eating behaviour, so you can plan changes accordingly. Your diary might look something like the one I have drawn up in Table 12.1. Alternatively, you mighht want to use a mobile app (see Resources):

Other behavioural strategies which are helpful include:

- Setting yourself realistic goals – One of the most common reasons people give up is because they set themselves too ambitious a target then feel they have 'failed'.
- Planning meals and snacks in advance rather than making last-minute choices; watch your portions; don't skip meals; try to limit eating to specific locations like your dining table.
- Paying attention when eating, rather than eat while doing other activities like watching TV or working. Look back at the mindfulness exercise for eating an orange in Chapter 6 – you can use this strategy to eat your whole meal mindfully.
- Managing cravings by delaying/distracting yourself with other activities and allowing yourself a range of healthy foods – rather than forbid anything in particular, have the occasional treat in moderation.
- Not weighing yourself too often – once a week is sufficient.
- Being self-compassionate – if you do have a lapse, don't beat yourself up about it. Forgive yourself and start again the next day with a positive mindset.
- Creating a supportive network – Partner up with someone to work on your changes together so you can spur each other on. Share your plan with friends and family so they can support you through times when you may be struggling and motivate you to keep going.

Date/Time/ Situation *What time of day was it? Where was I? What was I doing? Who was I with?*	**What did I eat and drink?** *List everything you ate-full meals as well as any snacks*	**Was your diet was balanced for this day? Why?/Why not?** *Think about the nutritional value of what you ate. Did you incorporate items from different food groups? You can look this up or use an app on your phone*	**Was it Emotional Eating?** *Was it a planned meal time? Was I hungry? Or was I bored, worried, anxious, upset, (or any other feeling)? Describe the feeling and rate it's intensity (0= lowest; 10-highest)*	**Reactions and Reflections on Emotional Eating** *What might have triggered it (e.g. stress/ relationship conflict)? Is there something significant happening in my life right now? Did I stop when I realised I was emotional eating? What helped me manage it? Did anything make it worse? What could I do instead of eating to cope with my feelings?*

TABLE 12.1 Food and Feelings Diary

Aches and pains in the joints

We probably all expect to get some aches in our muscles and joints as we age, and this might distract us from thinking it could be related to menopause. However, for many of us, musculo-skeletal aches and pains form a significant part of our menopausal experience. Up to 40% of all menopausal women in the UK are affected by joint pain.[3] Although we can get joint pain anywhere in the body, pain in the hips and knees in particular can cause difficulties in mobility and flexibility and can lead to longstanding injuries becoming more painful. This can have quite a debilitating effect on our life.

What causes joint pain?

A number of factors can contribute to joint pain, such as:

Weight gain – The extra weight we can put on during menopause may put increased strain on our joints, causing pain. Our knees are probably the most commonly affected joints. They are our largest joints and have to take a lot of pressure from our other connected body parts, supporting a large portion of our weight.

Reduced oestrogen levels – It is not fully known what causes perimenopausal joint pain, but experts believe that fluctuating hormones, particularly, falling oestrogen, may be a contributing factor. Oestrogen is thought to play a role in maintaining the fluid levels throughout the body. So, it keeps the joints lubricated, helping to protect them and reduce inflammation. As our oestrogen level drops, we are more prone to inflammation in our joints, causing aches and pains, and stiffness. Commonly affected joints include the hands, shoulders, knees and hips, although all joints can be affected.[4] As there is a significant drop in oestrogen at menopause, some of us may continue to experience joint pain in postmenopause. However, it can be difficult to know if the drop in oestrogen is always responsible for postmenopausal joint pain, as this period also coincides with increasing cases of age-related osteoarthritis (inflammation of the joints).[5] A decrease in oestrogen during perimenopause can also result in a loss in bone density. In severe cases, this can lead to osteoporosis, which is thinning of the bone causing them to become more fragile and break easily.[6]

Dehydration – Not drinking enough water and/or experiencing hot flushes and night sweats can make us dehydrated. This can exacerbate the effects of low oestrogen in our body, which in turn can lead to further joint pain. This may be why we might experience stiff joints in the morning after we have had night sweats. When we are dehydrated, it can also be harder for our kidneys to excrete excess uric acid, which can also make our joints sore and inflamed.

My meno moments

- As with other symptoms, I did not initially relate my joint pains to menopause. I had recovered from a knee injury from my teens and a weak ankle from my early 30s, which rarely troubled me. But more recently, I developed quite severe joint problems. Some mornings, I'd wake up and feel like I couldn't stretch out my arms without my elbows hurting, then not being able to put weight on my ankles when stepping out of bed and feeling my joints were too weak to walk down the stairs. Then there would be days when both my thumb joints were so painful that I couldn't lift a can of beans or open a jar. Having had scans and been told there is nothing physically wrong (no sign of arthritis), I was sent to a physiotherapist for advice on physical exercises to reduce the pain. Then, I read that muscle aches and joint pains are a common symptom in menopause.
- I recall a worrying moment on a wet autumnal day when I was trying to drive off in my car, and my knee suddenly 'clicked' when I pressed the accelerator pedal. I froze and couldn't push hard enough to get the car going. I had to sit in the car for about 10 minutes for the pain to ease before I felt okay to drive home. It made me think, what if I was on a hill – would I have rolled down not being able to control my car? I had already switched from a manual to an automatic car many years ago because of my existing knee problem, so now what, will I have to get a self-driving car? Then, that afternoon, I had to tell my 83-year-old mother that I couldn't manage the one-hour drive to go and see her because I didn't want to take the risk of getting caught out with my knee going into some sort of spasm while driving.
- I noticed that my joint pains have probably coincided with an increase in weight. I have never thought of myself as being slim, though looking back at old photos, I can see that I was well within the average weight range for my height. Over the years, I have gradually put on weight, especially after each pregnancy – around 6kg per child. From my mid–40s, a number of injuries and the joint pains led to me becoming less active. Then came all the sitting around working online during the Covid-19 lockdowns. In addition to that, I had heel pain from plantar fasciitis, so when walking was practically the only exercise we could do, the pain in my heels made it

hard to walk for very long. I attributed my weight gain to all these factors without realising that my hormonal fluctuations during perimenopause were also likely to be a contributing factor.

Coping strategies

Attitude of personal responsibility

Within my faith-based idea that nothing I own is actually mine as I pass through this transitory life, I see myself as being the guardian or custodian of my body. I have been blessed with and entrusted with this body. Reminding myself of this makes me try my best to do all that is in my power to take care of it. This does not mean that I blame myself for my weight gain or joint pain and have to beat myself up about it. Or that I don't seek treatment when needed. It just means that on a practical level, I need to take seriously the advice about living a healthy and balanced life and put in the effort to make simple lifestyle changes wherever I need to and can.

Nutrition, weight management and muscle mass

There are a number of food groups that have been suggested to be helpful for maintaining strong bones and preventing inflammation of the joints. As being heavier puts more pressure on our joints and muscles, potentially having a detrimental effect on them, managing our weight and trying to lose any excess will go a long way in reducing aches and pains. If you are trying to lose weight by cutting calories, one thing to be cautious of is that you are likely to be losing muscle mass too. If overdone, this could lead to impaired muscle function.[7] Research has shown that if you combine a reduced-calorie diet plan with strength-training exercises (such as lifting weights), it helps to lose fat around your midsection while preventing the loss of lean muscle which can occur with dieting alone.[8] The more muscle you have and the stronger your muscles are, the firmer your body will be, and the more energy you will have. It's best to seek the advice of a dietician to get up-to-date advice. You could check out the book 'Next Level' by exercise physiologist and nutrition scientist, Dr Stacy Sims. With her motto, 'women are not small men', she references research based on women's bodies for recommendations on nutrition and exercise during peri- and post-menopause (see Resources).

Keep exercise regular, consistent and varied

Try to avoid having sporadic bursts of activity followed by inactivity. You should build up your activity gradually, because if you push your body too hard, it can go into adrenal stress and disrupt the delicate hormonal balance in your body. Regular and consistent physical activity will not only strengthen muscles and aid mobility, it can also help you maintain a healthy weight, relieving any extra pressure on joints. You can engage in a range of physical activities and ideally during menopause you should incorporate two types of exercises which help build and maintain bone density: weight-bearing (which can be high impact or low impact) and muscle-strengthening (resistance) exercises, again being cautious not to put too much pressure on your joints. It would be ideal to get advice from a physiotherapist or a personal trainer for this or attend a gym to get advice on how best to do the exercises. And a reminder again, that it is best to consult your doctor for advice on what is safe and appropriate for you before you embark on a new exercise plan. Dr Sims' book mentioned above gives examples from athletes but less athletic women also report finding it very helpful.

From a psychological perspective, it is advisable to do activities that you actually enjoy in order to stay motivated. Take a look at the Balanced Lifestyle Log I shared in Chapter 7 and the table analogy to include physical exercise as one of the core elements of having a healthy lifestyle. If you have not already started to incorporate some physical activity into your weekly log, look for some gaps in the week where you can start doing this; then you can build up from there. You can progress slowly by increasing the frequency of your activity, or the intensity, or the duration. The aim is to do it gradually and at a pace that feels comfortable for you.

Don't stop; keep moving!

Just like we lose muscle mass, our bone strength also starts to decline as we age. Also, it can be hard to be motivated to exercise when we might not be sleeping well, feeling tired during the day, having hot flushes, joint pain and so on. One survey of physical activity in menopausal women found that 30% had become 'less active' during menopause and menopausal symptoms and low motivation for being active were among the reasons given.[9] This is just at a time when we need to be exercising *more* often to offset the changes in our heart health, bone density and muscle tone. It may sound counterintuitive to be exercising when our joints hurt, but numerous research studies have shown that bone loss can be slowed down by doing weight-bearing exercise. And some studies suggest that the stress put on the bone with this type of exercise stimulates extra deposits of calcium and pushes the bone-forming cells (osteoblasts) into action, thus forming more bone. This improves the strength and density of the bone.

I often had periods of time when I stopped exercising because I was worried about doing damage to already painful joints. But then I learnt that the way to improve joint pain was not to completely rest the joints but to keep them moderately activated. Implementing exercises targeted at the areas causing us pain can help ease the pain. It's best to do low impact exercises so we are putting less strain on the body while still strengthening the muscles that support our joints. I had pain in both knees but the left is always worse due to a previous injury, and sometimes I felt my ankles were also weak. In addition to that, I had the heel pain from plantar fasciitis. But I decided to invest in a comfortable pair of walking boots into which I inserted my custom-made heel inserts and took a graded approach by setting myself small targets of walking 20 minutes every day which amounted to about 5000 steps. When I was able to keep this up for a couple of weeks, I increased the duration of my walk and the steps. It is really motivating to have an app or smart watch to monitor your progress.

Sleep well

In combination with weight-bearing exercise, good bone health requires getting sufficient sleep. Studies have shown that unhealthy sleep duration – less than 6 hours or more than 10 hours – might contribute to reduced bone mass. So, maintaining a healthy sleep duration may be an effective approach to prevent bone loss.[10] (See Chapter 13 on sleep.) More research is required to determine which sleep/circadian disturbances are most detrimental to skeletal health, what the underlying mechanisms are and whether the impairments can be reversed.[11]

Stay hydrated

Drinking plenty of water helps to keep bones supple. Aim for 1.5–2 litres of plain water daily. You can give yourself prompts to increase your fluid intake. I find I drink more water when it is accessible to me, so when at home, I will have some whenever I walk past the fridge, for example. If going in to the clinic, I will take a bottle of water to drink on the journey, and refill it several times during the day. It is also advisable to limit your intake of coffee and tea as caffeine is a diuretic, so it makes your body lose water. Herbal teas are better. If you suffer night sweats and your joints feel sore in the mornings, try drinking a small glass of water an hour before going to bed.

Practical strategies

When your joints are hurting, there are a number of things you can try to ease the pain, such as placing a cold-compress on the location of pain, using a heated pad or hot water bottle, having a warm bath, doing some gentle stretching exercises, practising relaxation techniques and mindfulness (see the Appendix to locate these in previous chapters). There are also over-the-counter options to help reduce inflammation and painful joints, such as painkillers and anti-inflammatory gels and medication, which may be used with advice from the pharmacist.

Key points

Weight gain is caused by both ageing and menopausal hormone activity

Low impact exercises are best for strengthening muscles that support your joints

Good nutrition is crucial for joints and weight management.

Today I am grateful for:

Having managed to establish a good exercise routine

The space in my back room for doing my yoga and weights sessions

My plantar fasciitis has almost gone

Your turn:

List your **key learning points** from this chapter

List two or three things (big or small) you are **grateful for** right now

13 Poor Sleep and Insomnia

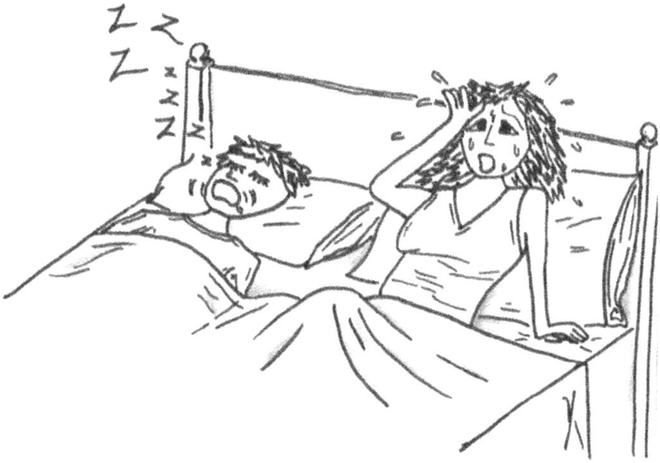

It cannot be over-emphasised how fundamental sleep is to our wellbeing. In fact, by now, I have mentioned sleep so much I wondered if I might get away with doing what the character Rita in Willy Russel's play 'Educating Rita'[1] does when her tutor sets her an essay question: 'Suggest how you would resolve the staging difficulties inherent in a production of Ibsen's Peer Gynt'. She responds with just one brief line on a piece of paper: 'Do it on the radio'. Well, for sleep, my line would be: Sleep – we need it! No ifs or buts about it!

We don't just need sleep for the obvious reason of rest but to support our immune system and repair our body, help heal physical wounds and reduce inflammation. Sleep can help us maintain a healthy weight by controlling our blood sugar level. It is also essential for our brain health and memory functioning, and it protects us from stress and depression. In terms of what is a good amount of sleep, although we often hear people say they should get seven hours of sleep per night, there is actually no given definition of what is a 'normal' number of hours. It depends on age and varies from person to person. It is more important to get good quality sleep rather than a certain number of hours.

Simply looking at the problems we experience when we do not sleep well, menopausal or not, tells us how crucial it is for us. Poor-quality sleep or sleep deprivation may be at the root of many health problems and can have significant knock-on effects on our life more generally. Ongoing lack of sleep can have an impact on our immune system and increases our risk of health conditions, such as high blood pressure, heart disease, diabetes, long-term pain, anxiety and depression. It can make us irritable and impulsive. It can leave us feeling exhausted and cause us to have trouble concentrating or focusing on tasks, which can have an impact on our work performance, or even put as at risk of accidents due to slowed down reaction times.

Sleep is yet another area where we are disproportionately affected when we are menopausal. Estimates suggest that between 9 and 15% of the general population have sleep problems, compared to as many as 63% of menopausal women struggling with their sleep.[2] Sleep disturbances are common throughout the menopausal transition, and we have mentioned numerous times already how the negative impact of the lack of sleep or poor-quality sleep crops up as a contributory factor in many symptoms during menopause.

It is, however, also common for women during the menopausal transition to have problems with sleep independent of these symptoms. Menopausal women most commonly report difficulty falling asleep, frequently waking up during the night and/or early-morning awakening and less restorative sleep (not feeling as rested on waking). The prevalence of sleep disorders has been found to increase as we age and progress along the menopausal journey, ranging from 39 to 47% in perimenopausal women and from 35 to 60% in postmenopausal women.[3] The range of these prevalence rates is likely down to the way it is measured, with self-reporting tending to lead to an under-estimation on some aspects of sleep and over-estimation on other aspects, compared to laboratory-based sleep studies.

If sleep problems persist, they may worsen and could lead to insomnia. The term 'insomnia' is used variably in research literature. In some, it seems to be used generically to refer to any difficulties with sleep; in others, it refers to longer term sleep problems; and in others, it is used as a more clinical definition. In order to be diagnosed with 'insomnia disorder', you would have 'a predominant complaint of dissatisfaction with sleep quantity or quality, associated with one (or more) of the following symptoms and conditions:

- difficulty initiating sleep (i.e., trouble falling asleep)
- difficulty maintaining sleep
- early-morning awakening with inability to return to sleep, for at least three nights per week, over at least three months'.

Also, the sleep difficulty would occur despite having adequate opportunity for sleep and cause clinically significant distress or impairment in areas of your daily functioning. And, it could not be explained as an effect of any other disorder or be attributable to the physiological effects of any substances like drugs or medication.[4] It is worth pointing out though that you don't need to experience the full criteria for insomnia disorder to be impacted by sleep difficulties.

What causes poor sleep and insomnia?

Hormonal imbalance – The changes in our hormone levels during the menopause affect many of our body's regular routines and rhythms. Oestrogen regulates hormones, such as serotonin and dopamine, which affect both mood and the sleep–wake cycle, so when oestrogen levels drop, it can have an impact on sleep. Increased levels of follicle-stimulating hormone (FSH), for example, has been linked to more disrupted sleep.[5] Also, when progesterone level drops, sleep may not come as easily because this hormone has calming, relaxing properties.

Secondary effects of other menopausal symptoms – The hormonal imbalances that cause symptoms, such as night sweats and dry itchy skin, can lead to disrupted

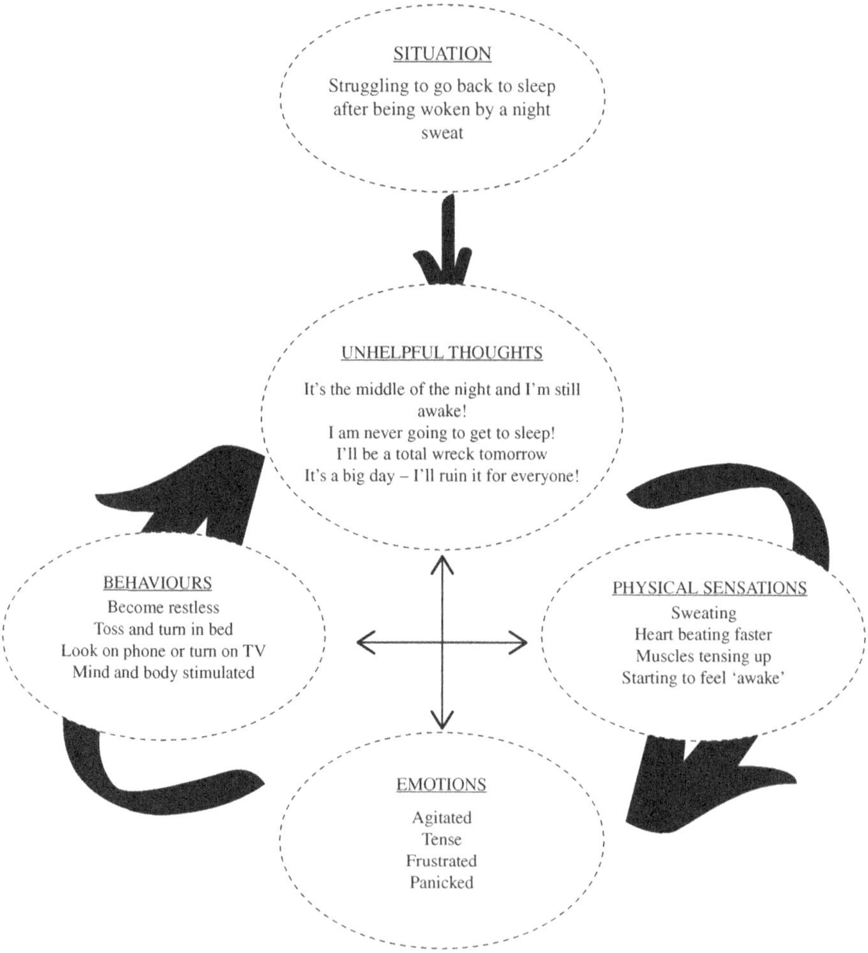

FIGURE 13.1 Vicious Cycle for Anxiety Related to Sleep

sleep or difficulty in falling asleep. When we have a night sweat, the body releases the stress hormone adrenaline – this stimulates our mind. We may become anxious and frustrated about not being able to sleep, which makes it more difficult for us to switch off and go back to sleep – another example of a vicious cycle (see Figure 13.1).

Ageing and other physiological effects – There are numerous other ways our sleep may be affected such as: our body making less of the 'sleep hormone' melatonin as we get older and an overactive bladder (due to decreased oestrogen level causing the bladder tissues to thin and lose tone) making us need to get up to use the bathroom at night.

Stress and mental health conditions – We looked at how the juggling of a multitude of tasks and responsibilities during our menopausal years causes stress and the impact of anxiety and low mood on our sleep in Chapter 5. There is a two-way relationship between sleep and mental health, in that one can be both a cause and consequence of the other. For example, poor sleep may create difficulties regulating emotions which, in turn, may leave you more vulnerable to depression. Depression is associated with sleep problems, such as shortening the amount of restorative slow wave sleep a person gets, and 75% of people with depression have trouble falling asleep or staying asleep.[6]

Impact of physical health problems – Sleep can be disrupted by many medical conditions, such as: asthma, chronic obstructive lung disease (COPD), sleep apnoea, heart disease and arthritis.

My meno moments

- Insomnia had been a companion of mine long before menopause showed up. Being a night owl does not work with the conventional time-tabling of work and school schedules. Having children and a 9–5 job meant I spent many years in a sort of haze after only getting a few hours' sleep per night. Ironically, I was regularly advising my clients on the importance of sleep and how to improve on it, while I was exhausted from sleep deprivation myself.
- Some years before I hit perimenopause, when I was extremely stressed at work and home, I woke up to the importance of sleep for my physical and mental health, as well as for my safety. During a spate of a few weeks, my sleep was so bad that I kept having little accidents. For example, when driving, I sometimes was not reacting quickly enough, such as hitting a bollard when reversing the car. This would be bad enough if I was alone in the car, but as a mother with a child in the car, this made me feel so much worse. These incidents made me realise I needed to pull my socks up

regarding my sleep routine. Of course, I knew what to do to improve my sleep, and every now and then, I would be determined to follow the advice I gave my clients. It did work and I would see improvements in my sleep and energy levels for a while. Unfortunately, old habits die hard, and after a few months, I'd somehow find myself back to those late nights and still having to get up early and feeling tired all day. I went back and forth like this for years until I finally did sort out my sleep.

- When my perimenopausal journey started, I was having a lot of trouble sleeping again though as usual I didn't link it to perimenopause; that is, until the night sweats showed up, waking me up two or three times a night. And again, I found a good night's sleep was not mine to be had. Now I went from being a regular insomniac to a perimenopausal insomniac. And this was so much worse because it was in conjunction with my other menopausal symptoms. I had difficulty getting up in the mornings and was tired driving to work. To cope, I started requesting later start times at work where I could. Then, when I had the privilege of working mostly for myself, I could finally arrange a time schedule that suited my body clock. Or so I told myself. This helped a bit but it was not a good solution because although I got up later, I didn't feel the restorative effects of sleep by the morning. My increased knowledge about the detrimental effects of poor sleep on my mind and body and seeing some signs of this eventually made me more determined to deal with it for good (see below). So now I am a recovered insomniac with the occasional nights of falling off the wagon.

Coping strategies

As insomnia can exist independent of, as well as during menopause, we might ask whether it should be treated differently when it is related to menopause? The treatment of menopausal sleep problems will depend on the cause, so ideally, to effectively manage sleep disorders in menopausal women, we should identify what might be causing it. However, this can be hard to ascertain because, as we have seen, there could be a number of factors contributing to the problem. Hence, there are a range of possible treatment options.

HRT and non-hormonal medication

If you and your doctor conclude that it is vasomotor symptoms that are causing your sleep problems, they may recommend HRT or another medication to reduce vasomotor symptoms (as discussed in Chapter 3), which should consequentially improve sleep. Your doctor will also advise that some medicines can actually cause insomnia, or if your insomnia is related to a medical condition or to a medicine you're already taking, they will advise how best to manage sleep problems.

Anxiety and stress management

If you are trying to address stress and a hectic lifestyle as the contributing factor, the usual rules of healthy living will apply to help you to sleep well. Try not to take unresolved issues and worries from the day to bed. Use the worry management techniques in Chapter 6 or problem-solving strategy in Chapter 9 during the day to resolve problems. Practice a positive mind-frame by writing down what you did achieve, what went well and what you are grateful for. You can also practice mindful breathing while lying in bed. (See Chapters 6 and 7.)

Cognitive behavioural approaches

Following on from what I have explained about CBT in previous chapters, this approach helps you to identify what's causing your sleep problems by looking at how your beliefs might affect your sleep and evaluating how you can manage the unhelpful thoughts and worries that could be keeping you awake. Then the focus is on developing good sleep habits and avoiding behaviours that might be preventing you from sleeping well. It is not a quick-fix – it takes time and effort to make it work. In some cases, a combination of sleep medication and CBT might be needed, especially until good sleep habits are established and sleep improves.

Cognitive strategies

You can use the noticing, challenging and cognitively restructuring strategies discussed in this book (see Chapters 6 and 7) to change your unhelpful thoughts related to sleep, come up with a different perspective of more helpful thoughts. For example:

UNHELPFUL THOUGHTS	HELPFUL THOUGHTS
I dread going to bed – I know I won't be able to sleep.	Even if it takes a while, I will fall asleep at some point. I will get some sleep if I let go and trust in my body's natural ability to sleep.
It's the middle of the night and I'm still awake! I won't be able to function properly tomorrow.	This has happened before. I did cope. I might be tired, so I will take it easy when I can, and I will be OK.

Behavioural strategies

There are numerous well researched and proven behavioural strategies which are effective for developing good sleep habits and resolving sleep problems as a long-term solution. Some of these ideas will seem really obvious, but like we've said before, we often don't do things we know are good for us, so a little reminder never hurts.

a. Stimulus control – When you struggle to fall asleep, you may lay awake tossing and turning and worrying about not sleeping. In this way, you condition yourself to associate your bed and bedroom with anxiety (conditioned arousal) and wakefulness. Stimulus control is aimed at breaking this conditioned association.
    - Use your bed only for sleeping or sexual activity. Avoid watching TV or using your laptop or phone once in bed. This helps your brain and body to associate your bed with sleeping and not wakefulness.
    - For the same reason as above, if you can't sleep, don't linger in bed. If you don't fall asleep, or wake in the night and can't go back to sleep within 20 minutes, get up and go into another room. Do something that won't stimulate your mind too much, like reading. Don't start watching something on a screen. Try not to watch the clock. Go back to bed when you start feeling sleepy.

b. Restricting unhelpful time in bed – Sometimes you might try really hard to get sleep, even going to bed earlier and/or lying in longer, but all you do is spend time lying awake. You might be worrying about whether you will get to sleep, stay asleep and (if you awaken) get back to sleep. One strategy is to reverse this process by limiting the time spent in bed to only the hours you will actually sleep. As a result of staying awake longer, your sleep drive builds up, and when you go to bed, you are more likely to fall asleep easily and stay asleep. As the quality of your sleep improves, you can gradually extend your time in bed until you get sufficient sleep.
    - Set yourself a consistent bedtime and wake time, and stick to them throughout the week (so no long lie-ins even at the weekend). This helps regulate your body's internal clock – the circadian rhythm – and improve the quality of your sleep.
    - If you end up not having slept well, don't be tempted to give yourself extra time in bed. Make sure you still get up at the normal time the next morning. You may feel a bit more tired than usual during the day, but by increasing your body's appetite for sleep, you'll get a better night's sleep the next night. This will put you back on track for sound sleep after that. Once your sleep improves, your time in bed will gradually increase.

c. Sleep hygiene – This is a guideline for addressing other factors that affect sleep, such as environmental conditions, use and timing of substance consumptions and physical activity.
   - Exercise regularly during the day. Don't over-exert yourself within two hours of going to bed.
   - Establish a bedtime routine – Start winding down about an hour before you plan to go to bed. For example, switch off and avoid screens; take a relaxing bath; do some light reading; or listen to some relaxing music.
   - Avoid or limit alcohol, nicotine, caffeine, fizzy drinks or chocolate, especially late in the day. Avoid large meals and beverages before bed. Avoid going to bed when you are too hungry or too full – a light snack before bed is OK.
   - Dress comfortably for bed in lightweight, preferably cotton sleepwear. Use light layers for bedding to avoid getting over-heated.
   - Establish a good sleep environment – Make your bedroom a comfortable and calming place to be in; ideally, it should be dimly lit or dark, quiet and cool but not cold.
   - Use breathing and relaxation techniques (see Chapter 6) to calm your mind and body before going to bed or to make you sleepy again if you wake up in the night.
   - If you are prone to night sweats waking you up in the night, get a change of clothes or towel ready before you go to bed to make it easier to go back to sleep quickly. To cool down, maybe open a window or go and stand on a cold bathroom floor.

The important thing to remember is to do these things consistently in order to build them up as habits. One of the strategies some people, including me, particularly struggle with, is the instruction to get out of bed when you can't sleep. It can be hard to leave your warm, comfortable bed after you wake up in the middle of the night. But, it is important to stick with it. To motivate you, see it as an investment in better sleep – maybe tonight is not so good, but you will be progressing towards better sleep on subsequent nights and building the habit of a good sleep pattern for the future. I would recommend 'Overcoming Insomnia' by Professor Colin Epsie as a good self-help guide using cognitive behavioural techniques (see Resources).

Keeping a sleep diary

Keeping a record of your habits and behaviours in relation to sleep may help you understand your sleep patterns better and notice areas of your daily routine that might not be helping. You can then try some simple changes like those suggested

Sleep Diary

Complete this diary each day for one or two weeks. Complete the shaded area just before going to bed, and the non-shaded area in the morning. **For ratings: 0= least, 10 = most**

Date/Day:							
How tired I felt during the day (0-10)							
How active I was during the day (0-10)							
Time spent outside in natural light?							
My mood rating during the day (0-10)							
Any naps during the day-number/duration?							
Any exercise within 4 hours of bed?							
Caffeine, alcohol, high-sugar foods within 4 hours of bed?							
Any TV or time on phone just before bed?							
Time I went to bed?							

TABLE 13.1 Sleep Diary

Any activity in bed – e.g. Read, TV, etc							
Time I put lights out							
Number of times I woke in the night							
Times I got out of bed-how long for?							
Time I woke up							
Total hours I slept							
Quality of sleep: I feel 0-10 (0 = exhausted; 10 = refreshed)							
Time I got out of bed							
Total hours spent in bed							
Additional notes: e.g. Stress/worry/night sweats?; sleeping pills?							

Suggestions for getting the most put of your sleep diary:

- Leave your sleep diary by your bed so you can fill it in before going to bed and when you wake up in the morning.
- Don't stress about being so accurate - an estimation of your sleep is fine, you don't have to know the exact number of times you wake us so don't try to remember it during the night as you don't want it to disrupt your sleep.
- Take a look at your daily habits (in the evening) and the quality of your sleep (in the morning) – Do you see any links between them? For example, did a behaviour such as drinking coffee or exercising too close to bedtime, lead to an outcome like poorer sleep or tiredness the next day?

TABLE 13.1 (Continued)

above to help improve the quality of your sleep. If you have tried some self-help strategies and are still struggling to sleep, you could share your sleep diary with your GP for further treatment advice. Further down the line, they might refer you to a specialist sleep clinic for assessment and treatment if necessary.

Your sleep diary might look like the one in Table 13.1. Alternatively, you may prefer to use digital resources, such as a fitness tracker or a health app to monitor your sleep. Though these might not always be 100% accurate, they can record relevant information, such as the quality of your sleep, which you can compare with your own observations. You could also try 'Sleepio', a NICE-recommended online sleep improvement programme based on the CBT approach.

CBT for insomnia (CBT-I)

This is a specific CBT-based treatment programme developed for the treatment of insomnia, which includes the cognitive behavioural strategies described above. It is comprised of the following components: psychoeducation about the connection between thoughts, feelings, behaviours, and sleep; stimulus control; sleep restriction; sleep hygiene; strategies to decrease arousal; and cognitive therapy. There is good evidence that CBT-I is effective in improving the quality and quantity of the sleep of those who complete the treatment, both from their own reporting and objective measurements. So, it is recommended as the first-line treatment of adults with insomnia.[7,8]

ACT for insomnia

Research also suggests that ACT approaches can be used to improve sleep and treat insomnia. For example, if you lie awake in bed worrying about not being able to sleep or thinking about other problems or worries, you might practice ACT techniques, like noticing (see Chapter 7) and thought defusion (see Chapter 6) to try and let go of these worries. Some studies have used only ACT to treat insomnia and other studies have incorporated ACT with other treatment approaches.[9] You can check out the *The Sleep Book* by Dr Guy Meadows if you are interested in the ACT approach (see Resources).

How I overcame my struggles with sleep

For many of us, dealing with insomnia or sleep problems in general can feel like a steep hurdle to overcome. I know it has been one of my biggest challenges. For example, I often enjoy doing things on a whim, and I hate to just stop what I am doing and go to bed because it's 'bedtime'. In Asian households when I was young, and even now in many homes, bedtime is a very loose concept. And I had never seriously given myself a bedtime as an adult. However, after years of having advised others about structure and routine, I recently really set my mind on following my own advice using the cognitive behavioural strategies described above.

First, I worked on getting a structure to my day and week and established some routines. I made sure I did some physical activity every day. I went to bed earlier each day in increments of 15 minutes – so where I had been going to bed at 2 a.m., I went to bed at 1.45 a.m. for a couple of nights, then 1.30 a.m. for another couple of nights and so on until I reached a bedtime of 12.30 a.m., which I felt was a relatively reasonable time for me. In order to achieve this, I had to change a number of my bad habits – I had to avoid starting 'just another episode of ...' on TV, or 'just finish off a bit of work to save time tomorrow' or sort out a basket of laundry for putting in the washing machine in the morning. And I had to start winding down from about an hour before the time I was due to go to bed. Regarding my waking up time, for some reason, I would always wake at around 9 a.m. even when I went to bed at 3 a.m. But then I had this habit of staying in bed, reaching for my phone and checking my messages and emails for another half hour or even an hour at times. So, I had to force myself to stop this habit, set my alarm for 8.30 a.m. and get out of bed as soon as the alarm went. I did this by placing my phone just out of arms reach so that I would have to get up to turn the alarm off. Of course, leaving the phone in another room would have been even better, but I used the excuse that I needed it for the alarm, having rejected the separate alarm clock my husband had bought me.

So, you might have calculated that 12.30 a.m. to 8.30 a.m. would amount to eight hours of sleep. But I am not someone who falls asleep as soon as my head hits the pillow. I would usually read for a bit, then find it hard to switch off. That's partly why my sleep problems are worse when I have a lot to think about, whether due to stress or excitement. On nights when I couldn't sleep, I reminded myself about the strategies I described above, and I really had to push myself to get out of bed, go downstairs and quietly read for a while until I felt sleepy and could return to bed. So, I probably actually got around seven hours' sleep, which for me is sufficient to feel rested for the next day. It took me about six weeks to develop a sleep routine that works well for me now. There are just two aspects of being a Muslim that can disrupt my sleep and I have to manage: (1) Waking up for the dawn prayer – it only takes a few minutes to get up and do, but I can find it hard to get back to sleep, though my body is getting used to it; (2) During Ramadan – when I have to get up to eat and pray at dawn, fast until sunset and can feel lethargic during the day. Ramadan does mess up my system for a month and can take me another month afterwards to fix. But I accept that, because it means I am aligned with my values of faith and worship, and I appreciate the physical benefits of fasting and spiritual benefits I reap from those committed actions.

Key points

Getting good quality sleep is crucial for our physical and mental wellbeing

Even small lifestyle changes help towards developing good sleep

Today I am grateful for:

I finally sorted out my sleep routine!

Having more energy during the day

Improved focus and concentration

Your turn:

List your **key learning points** from this chapter

List two or three things (big or small) you are **grateful for** right now

Part III

Impacts and Wider Perspectives

14 Impacts on Self-Identity and Relationships

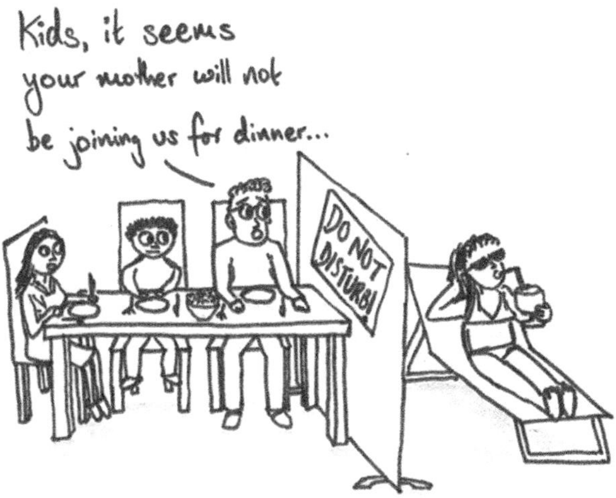
Kids, it seems your mother will not be joining us for dinner...
DO NOT DISTURB!

It's not just physically and mentally that menopause affects us. It can have deeper and more far-reaching impacts on our life. Whether we have a relatively brief and smooth menopause transition period or a prolonged and difficult journey, it will change us and the way we relate to others.

Is it menopause or am I just getting old?

In South-Asian cultures, we don't call adults who are of the same generation as our parents by their names – we call them 'uncle' or 'auntie'. Here, the term 'auntie' might be seen as equivalent to the term 'women of a certain age' in the West referring to 'middle-aged women' – an age that it is considered impolite to specify with a number. My friends and I used to laugh at how 'the aunties', that is, our mums and their friends, would always be complaining about their physical ailments when they got together. But in the last few years, we started to find ourselves talking about our heavy periods, how we'd started forgetting things, how our knees hurt, our numerous hospital appointments and so on. It suddenly dawned on us we were becoming the aunties ourselves!

Of course, there is no denying that as we age, in addition to developing wrinkles, greying hair and potentially diminished eyesight and hearing, we do start experiencing little niggles within our body. And the chances of developing more serious health conditions are increased. With some overlaps in symptoms, it can also be hard to know whether those symptoms are due to menopause or a part of the natural ageing process. For example, these are some of the changes that happen with ageing that you might experience during menopause:[1]

- *Bones, joints and muscles* – Our bones tend to shrink in size and density, are weakened and become more susceptible to fracture. Muscles tend to lose strength, endurance and flexibility.
- *Memory and thinking skills* – Our brain's capacity gradually declines, so we can experience problems with cognitive functioning and memory – for example, being forgetful or not as adept at multitasking as we might have been before.
- *Skin changes* – Our skin becomes thinner, less elastic and more fragile. The fatty tissue just below the skin reduces, less natural oils are produced, so our skin becomes drier.
- *Weight* – Our metabolism slows down, and we also tend to be less active. So, if we continue to eat the same as usual, we will gain weight.
- *Sexuality* – Our sexual desire and activity might also change. Illness or medication might impact on our ability to enjoy sex. Vaginal dryness can make sex uncomfortable.
- *Bladder and urinary tract* – Our bladder may become less elastic and the bladder muscles and pelvic floor muscles may become weaker. This can cause us to feel the need to urinate more often and maybe have problems with bladder control.

So, unless we've gone into early menopause, when we experience overlapping symptoms like these, we will need the help of our doctor to work out what the underlying cause might be and how best to approach the management of symptoms.

Change to sense of self– Who am I now?

Along with the physical changes, we are changing in other ways too. Going through menopause might trigger us to reflect on our life so far and review our hopes and aspirations. Have we achieved what we hoped and planned to? Are we happy with who we have become? Depending on our reflections, we may feel satisfaction and/ or disappointment. The process of reflection may even feel a little disconcerting, especially if we feel a sense of loss for missed opportunities. And while also battling with menopausal symptoms, it can all feel quite overwhelming.

Menopause occurs at a time in our life when we may also be going through lots of other stressful events and are probably busier than we've ever been. We might be juggling our careers with a family of children as young as toddlers or teenagers about to leave home. At the same time, we may also find ourselves either solely responsible or having shared responsibility for care of our ageing parents. We may be happily single or looking for a partner. Or if married or living with a partner, we need to be giving our attention to that relationship too. In fact, depending on our circumstances, trying to balance our many responsibilities can feel overwhelming at times. And when significant events in life occur – such as the death of an elderly parent, illness of a partner, marriage of a son or daughter, birth of a grandchild – our menopausal symptoms might pale into insignificance, as some women report.[2]

With so much going on, it can be easy to neglect yourself, forget who 'you' are and find very little time to look after yourself. I liked this reflection from one woman taking part in a qualitative research study: 'You seem to spend that first half of your life trying to be fairly perfect, you try to fit that mould and what you may see as the right sort of thing by doing all the right things and keeping everyone happy because that's a big thing and always trying to keep things in balance. Maybe you get to 50 and you think, well bugger it, you've done all that work and all that effort and you think, gee have I ever really given myself enough pleasure and consideration'.[3]

Loss of periods, loss of fertility

The most obvious change that menopause brings is of course the physical aspect of no longer having periods. Many women may feel liberated from the monthly inconvenience of it. And it may especially be a welcome relief if you've been used to very heavy and erratic periods in your premenopausal or perimenopausal years. But others may miss the cycles of periods and can feel a bit disorientated without them or can feel like they've lost their femininity without them.

Then, there is the more emotional aspect of the loss of fertility that reaching menopause brings. No longer being able to have children can mean different things to different women and can trigger very mixed feelings in some. If you wanted children or hadn't even thought about it yet and got diagnosed with early menopause, you may feel devastated by the loss of the choice to have them. Though there may be hope in terms of fostering, adoption and, for some, fertility treatment options, you might still feel a bit short-changed by mother nature. Or perhaps you wanted children but never got around to it for whatever reason, you might have had the thought at the back of your mind that it's still possible. Until menopause hits. Then, you can feel sad and may regret your decisions, maybe even ruminate about past relationships which might have led to children. So, then you have to accept the inevitable and may find yourself grieving the children you never had. You may see friends' or relatives' children growing up or see them becoming grandparents and again feel a sense of loss.

Even if you have children and thought you had completed your family by the time you reach menopause, you might be surprised by a feeling of a sense of loss when you can't have any more. For example, I have a friend who has three sons, and reaching menopause at 45, had a difficult time accepting that she would no longer be able to try for a daughter. If you never particularly wanted to have children, you may have no issue with the loss of fertility or you might feel a sense of the lost opportunity to change your mind.

The loss of fertility can also bring with it an increased awareness of ageing – signalling the end of your youthful years and maybe feeling a loss of femininity – as well as remind you of your mortality.

My meno moments

- One summer evening, I found myself outside a party hall with two other women because we all found it far too hot and noisy inside. We were all in our 50s, so the conversation quite quickly became personal and we shared menopause stories. We all agreed that for us the worst symptom was brain fog because of the way it affects our sense of who we thought we were. We were intelligent, professional women in positions of responsibility, who had worked hard to get to where we were. But now we keep getting stuck trying to find words we know.
- I have had times when I felt I had lost myself in the mist of all the brain fog. I knew I was fairly articulate and was told so by others, but what I always admired and wanted to be when I grew up was eloquent (think Maya Angelou). Now, when my brain fog is at its worst, I have to applaud myself for just being able to string a sentence together, never mind doing it stylishly! Now, I lament the good-enough articulate me with no room to hanker after eloquence. On bad days, I really don't like this dithery 'auntie' that I expect others see. Then, I may have a good day at work – for example, in a meeting I might retrieve words that I actually want rather than making do with a simpler alternative or make cogent arguments and clear decisions. Or, I'll be pleased with myself for quickly making a clever remark or joke that my family or friends enjoy. This will give me a glimpse of my old self and remind me I haven't lost myself completely.

Coping strategies

Allowing yourself to slow down and stop trying to do it all

There were many a times I was called a 'Supermum' in the school playground. And I'm sure I felt proud of that at the time. Like when I'd turn up on World Book Day with my child in a costume I'd sewn overnight, then rushing off to work with a report I'd finished within the deadline. I didn't acknowledge at the time how hard it was to keep it all going. Then, one day at a wedding, a throw-away remark by a distant relative led me to look more closely at myself. After the usual, 'how are you, haven't seen you in ages …' she chirpily said, 'Oh, you're not still doing all that work lark, are you!?' I was at a particularly stressful time in life and I remember feeling quite perturbed, my instant thought being, 'Huh, you can talk, all you do is stay at home having babies and cooking'. But later, I started to reflect on her words – perhaps she had the right idea, perhaps life would be easier if I had chosen to *either* be a stay-at-home-mum *or* a career woman. Why was I killing myself trying to do it all. Being brought up by a mother who believed her whole existence was about motherhood and caring for her family, she instilled in me the idea that I should be as devoted. But I had also had an ambitious father who encouraged education and professional pursuits, and given that he was ahead of his time in treating me as equal to my brothers in that matter, I had to honour that too.

I have never regretted any of my choices, and I do think it is possible to combine work and parenting well. Besides, for many women, it is not even a lifestyle choice but necessary for family economics. But at that time, I was a mother of two and doing three part-time jobs with a couple of voluntary roles on the side. This was not planned – I'd started my main job part time to fit around my family, but then taken on the other posts when they came along because they interested me, and I enjoyed them. I told myself they were 'only part-time' though they often added up to more than a full-time working week. But those words did get me thinking that something had to give – I needed to create some breathing space for myself. It triggered me to take a sabbatical from my main job for a year, then not going back.

And now, I simply cannot manage to do half as much as I used to do in my 30s and 40s. Whether it's down to ageing or the menopause, I don't know. But perhaps our menopausal symptoms might be a sort of wake-up call, nature's way of helping us pull in the reins and reset ourselves as we go into our older years.

In order to get the reflective space needed to think about your values and passions, you need to give yourself permission to slow down a little and take pauses from the daily grind of tasks. This is easier said than done because you might feel that everything you are doing is necessary and you are the only one who can do them. But in order to carve out a little time for yourself, it's worth taking the 'risk' and cutting down on a few things or delegating to others at work or home. Look back at the 'noticing' exercise in Chapter 7 to tune in to yourself when you feel overwhelmed, and ask yourself what thoughts come to mind that may be driving you to take on too much or set your expectations too high. (Also see the 're-evaluating your load' section in Chapter 6).

Adopting an 'I'm worth it' attitude

Women generally tend to take on caring roles, and over time they can end up neglecting themselves. There are only so many hours in a day and only so much energy you can muster, so by the time you've sorted everyone else out, you can be too exhausted to do something for yourself. Many of the women I have worked with over the years have needed help to recognise that they too deserve care and attention, and that doing things for themselves is not selfish or self-indulgent. I've had to work on this myself too. In fact, looking after yourself will benefit those you care for too. If you run yourself down, you won't be in a position to help anyone. After all, as is commonly said, 'you can't pour from an empty cup'. So, you need to give yourself permission to do things that will make you feel good, and once you believe you *deserve* it, you *will* somehow find the time.

Don't be afraid to take time for yourself or ask for help in getting it. For example, you may decide that if you had 20 minutes to meditate or for a soak in the bath, it would really help your stress levels, which in turn will help reduce menopausal symptoms. But then, you just can't find the time as there is so much to do when you get home from work. You could have a chat with your partner to explain why you need this time and negotiate how they might do a few tasks, or if you are caring for children or elderly parents alone, you could explain that you need some time to do something important for you and give them something to get on with on their own. And if your children are old enough, you shouldn't feel guilty about giving them little responsibilities and reduce some of the load on yourself. You could use the 'Balanced Lifestyle Log' in Chapter 9 as an activity diary for the whole family and in that enter some slots where other family members do certain regular chores and you have some 'me-time' – preferably away from home so you don't get dragged into their tasks!

Finding yourself again

It will be good for your sense of self-worth to try and 'find yourself' again under the rubble of the midlife chaos. You need to make time to first look after yourself physically, then to work out what you want from life, what gives you joy and what you are passionate about. This is crucial for your psychological and emotional health. You can look at the values section in Chapter 9 to try and work out what is meaningful to you and gives you a sense of purpose in life. For example, one of my key values is education, but I realised I had got so busy 'doing', I hadn't engaged in any 'new learning' for a while. However, I also felt I didn't have the capacity to take on too much. So, I have just been watching short courses on online on various topics of interest.

Count your blessings

If you find yourself ruminating over the past and feeling a sense of loss for how things didn't work out as you wished or expected, or what you didn't manage to do or achieve in life, it helps to try and build a habit of noticing and reflecting on things that *did* go well or what you *have* achieved, rather than focus on when things go wrong. Think about it, how often do we say, 'It turned out to be a good day today' compared to 'I had such a horrible day … (listing all the things that bothered us)'. Practising gratitude makes us thankful and less prone to complaining about what is missing in our life (see Chapter 7).

Impacts on our relationships

'Uh, don't talk to me about menopause. Menopause cost me my marriage!'

That was the reaction of a health professional I went to see when I queried whether my ailments might be related to menopause. Then, rather unprofessionally, he went on to tell me how his 'sweet-natured wife' with whom he was 'still in love' had turned into a 'monster' over the past couple of years. Then she left him and 'found herself another man within a few months'. With no encouragement from me (after all, I was the patient in this scenario), he went on to tell me his woes, which were obviously fresh, and even more so at each of my treatment sessions. He knew I was a psychologist, because I had to put my occupation on the registration form. I wished I'd lied! I assumed his wife had taken his sense of humour with her too, as he didn't stop after I said at the end of one session, 'I think *I* should be invoicing *you* for this one!'

His story made me think of possible scenarios: (1) perhaps it was a difficult relationship for any number of reasons and he's just blaming it all on his wife and her hormones; (2) maybe she was going through the menopause and neither of them knew how to manage it, resulting in the relationship becoming the 'casualty'; or (3) it was a combination of both those things. If menopause-related, it would highlight how it is not only women who need to be prepared for it, but also those with whom they share their lives. We might be the ones with the immediate impacts, but those around us are also affected.

In the UK, the highest divorce rate in opposite-sex couples is in the 45 to 49 years age range. And the divorce rate for those aged 55 and over – dubbed 'grey divorce' – has more than doubled since 1990.[4] Now we can't assume this is a menopausal fallout, as there may be many factors at play leading to these statistics, and we would need further research to show potential causal links. But the fact that it does coincide with the time when women are going through the turbulence of menopause warrants investigation in this area. It's also worth noting that nearly two-thirds of divorces are petitioned by women.[4] It might be worth considering what the instigating factors might be for women. Perhaps a sense of lack of support during this difficult time? Perhaps a sense of feeling empowered to move on in their lives in a new direction? It may also be a time when they do some soul-searching, reflect on their life and perhaps decide that some sort of change needs to happen. This is not necessarily just menopause-related but may also be an awakening about their mortality and reviewing their hopes and aspirations in life.

'We've come a long, long way together. Through the hard times and the good …'[5]

By the time we hit perimenopause, it's likely we have been in our relationship for some time. And even if we are in a fairly new relationship, we are not the same as we were in our youth. For both men and women, our bodies are not the same, and we will have emotional baggage either from being together or our individual baggage brought from previous relationships. Anyone in a long-term relationship will tell you it takes a lot of work. At a friends' get-together recently, someone mentioning the longevity of our union commented on how 'lucky' we were to have found each other and been together so long. It was perhaps because we weren't in the best mood with each in that instance that my husband and I both looked at each other irritated, as if to say, 'what's luck got to do with it!?' The reality is that sustaining a long-term relationship requires more than love – it's about effort, perseverance and digging deep to find your empathic best.

So, how do we navigate our middle-aged years together? There will be a need for sharing, understanding and compassion, both towards ourselves and our partners who are living with this too – an attitude of mutual support. In a survey of male partners (described further below), most men (70%) observed a negative impact of menopausal symptoms on their partner. But interestingly, slightly more (77%) thought it impacted on themselves. And just over half thought there was an impact on the relationship.[6]

And when we see that our partners of a similar age may be going through their own challenges (see below), there's room for empathy in both directions. We have to start, of course, by normalising the topic of menopause so that it becomes easier to talk about, as it seems that's not even happening enough among partners and married couples.

So, what do men know about menopause?

I was not able to find much in the way of research regarding men's knowledge and attitude towards menopause. In the 2019 MATE survey sent to 1,356 men, mostly aged between 50 and 69 years, with female partners aged between 45 and 64 years old, they were asked about their perceptions and attitudes towards menopause; 450 of them (33%) responded.[6] When asked what types of symptoms women typically experience when going through menopause, 55% said hot flushes/sweating and 44% said mood swings. Other symptoms they mentioned were low libido, irritability and depression/sadness, weight gain/bloating, night sweats, low energy and trouble sleeping. And when asked how they would describe menopause to other men, they described the irrational or emotional mood of their partners (22%) followed by hormonal change (21%). They also mentioned physical/biological/chemical changes (10%), not being able to have children (13%), not having menstrual cycles (12%) and change in sex drive (7%). It's a positive sign that there is some awareness of menopause among men though the survey did find that they did not consistently relate the symptoms to menopause and lacked knowledge about specific treatments. Like women, they could do with further information and education to improve on understanding and being supportive towards their partner, which can only be beneficial for the relationship.

Is my partner going through something too?

Male partners – Although women and men go through hormonal changes as they age, there are differences in how this occurs. During menopause, women experience a dramatic drop in hormone production over a relatively short period of time. In men, the production of testosterone and other hormones is more of a gradual decline, over a period of many years. A man's testosterone levels decline on average about 1% per year from around the age of 30 to 40, and this can often go unnoticed and not cause any symptoms. Most older men still have testosterone levels within the normal range, with only an estimated 10–25% having levels considered to be low.[7] This gradual decline of testosterone levels is called late-onset hypogonadism or age-related low testosterone. You might see the term 'male menopause' (or 'andropause') used generically to try to equate men's experience to that of women, but from a scientific or clinical perspective, this is unhelpful. It suggests a sudden drop in sex hormones, such as that occuring in women in perimenopause, which is not the case.

But, with a view to understanding what our partners may be going through at the same time us as, it is worth noting that these are the common symptoms men might experience from their late 40s to early 50s:

- reduced libido and sexual activity
- decrease in spontaneous erections or erectile dysfunction
- mood swings and irritability or depression
- reduced muscle bulk and strength and/or low bone mineral density
- increased body fat and unbalanced fat redistribution
- increased sleepiness or sleep problems (insomnia) or fatigue
- poor concentration and difficulties with short-term memory
- decreased energy, motivation and confidence

There is also not necessarily a clear link between the drop in testosterone levels and symptoms experienced by older men. They may not be associated with low testosterone at all, but attributable to other factors, such as age, obesity, lifestyle choices, psychological problems, medication use or other conditions. For example, erectile dysfunction may be caused by smoking or heart problems, as well as coinciding with psychological issues.

I have noticed my husband going through some of the symptoms described above – such as forgetfulness (e.g., leaving the front door open at night!). The other day, we had a shared experience of brain fog when he was going to pick up pizza and called to ask what I wanted on mine. I said, 'I'll have a vegetarian one but no mushroom and none of those ... what are they called, that you got last time ...? You know, they look like peppercorns ... why can't you help me ...?' His response, 'I know what you mean, but I can't remember either'. When he got to the restaurant, he realised, I was talking about capers. It can be upsetting to realise that you are getting old, and it can be just as sad to watch your partner getting old in front of your eyes too.

Female partners – Depending on their age, they may not have embarked on the menopause journey or may also be peri- or post-menopausal. As we know, each woman's experience is different, so if you are both going through it at the same time, each may or may not appreciate the other's difficulties. So, of course, communication is key.

Psychosexual issues

Sexual difficulties can occur at any time in an intimate relationship. During menopause, it is usually both a physiological and a psychological issue. The many physical and emotional changes we are experiencing during this transition are likely to have an impact on how we relate to our partner during our most intimate moments. Thinning, loss of lubrication and irritation of the vulva and vaginal tissue can cause discomfort during sex. We may be tired from sleep disturbances or insomnia and have reduced arousal. These symptoms can make us want to be left alone and generally not be in the mood for nights of passion. If not addressed, this may cause tension in the relationship. Alternatively, I have also heard some women report that their libido has increased during menopause and their partner may either be very pleased about this or dread it if their own libido is not so high. So, both partners will need to be understanding of the others' needs and make adjustments and perhaps even go on a journey of discovering new ways of enjoying intimacy.

'Dad, Dad, Mum's gone mad!'

If we have children while going through menopause, they may be anywhere in age from toddlers to teens or young adults. Younger children are unlikely to understand what's happening and may get confused by some of mum's menopause-related moods or actions. And perhaps the most difficult to manage will be toddlers (with all that *energy*!) and teenagers. As the average age at which a woman has her first child is 30.9 years,[8] her children are most likely to be in their teens when she is in perimenopause. The co-existence of puberty and menopause can feel like a whirlwind of hormones in the house – with all that emotional angst and identity crisis all around. And for the mother–teenage daughter relationship, there can be mixed hormonal responses, such as proudly watching your daughter blossom into a beautiful young woman, while at the same time lamenting the loss of your own youthfulness. A tough gig indeed!

One of my friends was describing her mood swings and the impact on her family: in a fluster of cooking after a long day at work, and with her hands occupied, she had asked her teenage son to fetch her a colander from the kitchen cupboard. Not knowing what exactly that was, he brought her a bowl; she told him that wasn't it, and it had holes in it. He then brought her a cheese grater. Irritated by this, she went to the cupboard and got the colander herself and almost went to hit him with it saying, 'that's a colander!'. Her son was shocked and ran to his father, saying, 'Dad, Dad, Mum's gone mad!'. Never having done anything like this before, she suddenly realised how far removed from 'herself' she had become, triggering her to make an appointment with her GP to discuss HRT which she'd been deliberating over for months.

And if the kids have left home, there can be a difficult period of adjustment for both parents (referred to as the 'empty nest syndrome'), which has the potential to bring out unresolved issues in the couple's relationship too. It's probably more common for the absence of children in the home to be felt more by mothers, as they may have been more involved in childcare and domestic chores. 'Losing' or rather 'letting go' of your children can be quite a heart-wrenching process and leave you re-thinking your purpose in life. As the children fly the nest, you need to find other ways to fill the gap, and do your own thing.

Coping strategies

Talk about it!

Communication is the key to success in all relationships, personal or otherwise. One of the most common causes of relationship breakdown is lack of communication. Our partners need to understand the changes we are going through both physically and emotionally, not only to be supportive, but also to maintain a healthy relationship. But we have a responsibility here too. We can't expect people to just understand, especially when sometimes we don't even understand it ourselves. We hardly recognise ourselves anymore, so it is likely our partner, children, friends and colleagues don't quite understand this new version of us either. So, it's important to share our experiences with those close to us.

Of course, with children, the language we use and how much we explain will depend on their age and developmental stage. But, it is still better to give them some information rather than trying to hide our symptoms from them. It's usually obvious there's something going on, and they will try to make their own sense of it, which may lead to the wrong conclusion and cause unnecessary anxiety and worry. It has been announced that students will now be taught about the menopause in sex and relationship lessons at secondary school as part of the UK curriculum.[9] So, this can be an opportunity to check with teenagers what they are being taught and start conversations at home so they understand what is happening for mum. Especially for teenagers, discussions about hormonal changes can be helpful to talk about in relation to what they are experiencing at their end too.

Turn to the sisterhood

If there's anyone who's going to really understand what we are going through, it will be our sisters in menopause. But remember we may have also got to a point where we won't put up with relationships that are emotionally draining and not mutually supportive. So, what we need is good company – a few good friends who know and accept us as we are and give us the reassurance and support we need. And we will also feel good to be able to give the same back. If we are lucky enough to have the bonds of existing long-term friendships that's great, but it's also never too late to develop new friendships if we are open to it. If you want to see a positive portrayal of older women and the bond of a lifelong friendship, I can recommend watching a film called 'Nyad' (2023).

Keeping intimacy going

Menopause does not have to spell the end of your sex life. The physiological symptoms can be treated with vaginal oestrogen and over-the-counter vaginal moisturisers or lubricants, for example. As for the psychological issues, the first step is to talk about it with your partner so you work through some of the challenges together. You might re-frame what a meaningful sex life is to you, rather than what you might think is 'expected' or the norm. Simply being affectionate can make you feel connected to your body and close to your partner. You might also have fun exploring what currently feels pleasurable with flirting, playfulness, new sexual experiences and being mindful during sexual activity. Also, at this age, it doesn't have to be spontaneous – you can schedule in times to be intimate. As I heard clinical psychologist, Dr Karen Gurney, say about sex within long-term relationships in a recent podcast, 'sexual relationships need to be able to flex and allow for growth'. You may want to check out her book, *Mind the Gap* (see Resources).

Couples therapy or psychosexual counselling

If there are relationship issues that have been left unresolved, that will also have an impact on your capacity for intimacy on an emotional level. If you are both experiencing difficulties simultaneously, you might lack compassion for each other. You might have drifted apart and need to learn to re-connect or re-negotiate the terms of the relationship. Sometimes this can be hard to do alone as you may be stuck in unhelpful patterns in your communication style, so seeking out support from professions will help.

Key points

Things may seem a bit cloudy at the moment, but you are still *you*

Give yourself permission to focus on yourself – make time for self-care

Let those close to you know what's going on for you

Today I am grateful for:

Developing the confidence to be *me* – an ongoing journey

All my close relationships

My communication, and more importantly, listening and reflecting skills

Your turn:

List your **key learning points** from this chapter

List two or three things (big or small) you are **grateful for** right now

15 Menopause at Work: Impacts and Adjustments

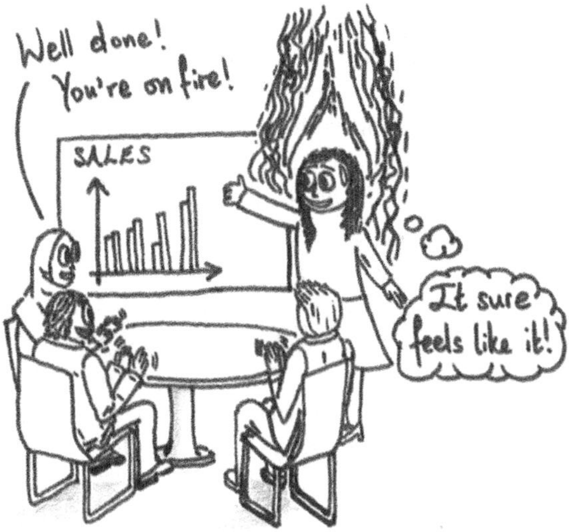
Well done! You're on fire!
SALES
It sure feels like it!

At the time of writing, there are 15.7 million women working in the UK[1] – that's 47% of the workforce. Of these, around 4.5 million are within the usual menopausal age of 50–64 years.[1] Considering that many women go into early menopause and experience perimenopausal symptoms for years beforehand, the number of the workforce potentially impacted by the menopause is significantly higher. This number will only increase as the UK state pension age is set to rise to 67 by 2028 and 68 by 2046.[2] And the current (and potentially ongoing for some time) cost-of-living crisis is possibly not going to make it easy for many women to leave employment as early as they may want to. So, the impact of menopause in the workplace needs serious consideration.

In most careers, it takes a good number of years to become established and work your way up to a senior position. So, we are likely to be around our mid-40s and 50s when this happens. Then, just as we are feeling confident in our skills and experience at work and are likely to be in a highly valued position after years of building our careers – often having sacrificed time for ourselves and our families – we can suddenly start to struggle with it because of the menopausal mayhem. That is not to say that menopause makes us incompetent in our roles, but that it throws even more challenges than we are already used to as women in the workplace and ones we were probably not prepared for. So, we can sometimes start doubting ourselves and perhaps ask, '*Can I still do my job?*'.

In fact, research has shown that around a quarter of working women have contemplated leaving their jobs because of the difficulties of trying to manage their menopausal symptoms on top of work and other life stressors.[3] The Fawcett Society, a women's rights charity, conducted what they describe as the largest representative survey of menopausal women conducted in the UK. Regarding the impact of menopause on work, they found 44% of women said their ability to work (currently and in the past) had been affected, 52% said they had lost confidence; 14% had reduced their hours at work, 14% had gone part-time and 8% had not applied for promotion. They also reported that 1 in 10 women had actually left a job due to menopausal symptoms (rising to 22% for disabled women).[4] There have been similar statistics reported for working women in USA and Australia.[5]

What these statistics demonstrate is that there is a significant number of women who are not being supported at work during their menopausal transition. It is also costly to the economy and employers when women need to take days off work due to symptoms. And for those who give up their jobs due to the lack of support, it is a loss to them and a loss to society, as these are skilled and experienced women leaving the workforce. It can also be costly for employers to replace a woman in her 50s who has left a senior position. If employers start to acknowledge the impact of menopause and make the necessary adjustments, this is potentially preventable and makes economic sense for them *even* if they were not particularly concerned about women's wellbeing.

Some menopause and work facts (UK):[3]

- 14 million working days are lost to menopause annually.
- Women of menopausal age are the fastest growing working demographic in the UK.
- One in four women consider leaving work due to the menopause.
- Women of menopausal age are often at the peak of their career.
- The cost of replacing trained employees places significant strain on businesses.

How does menopause show up at work?

As we have seen, menopause can have significant impacts on all aspects of our lives, so of course, that will include our working lives. Although some women might have the option of changing careers or reducing hours, for most, this will not be an option. So, ways need to be found for us to function well at work while effectively managing menopausal symptoms. As we also know, the menopause transition for many women is not a short-lived experience but can go on for a significant amount of time (between 2 and 10 years, with an average of 7 years), so appropriate long-term adjustments at work are necessary. Here are just a few ways in which some of the common symptoms of menopause might impact us at work:

- Heavy and painful periods – can make us feel tired and weak and need us to visit the loo more frequently or in a rush, which can be difficult during work interactions
- Hot flushes – can be physically uncomfortable, making us feel anxious and distressed
- Brain fog – can make us feel embarrassed and anxious when we cannot retrieve words during communication or slow us down in our work when we cannot focus or lose concentration
- Fatigue and low mood – can impact on our productivity, communication and relationships with colleagues

There are many factors that can make menopause symptoms harder to manage in the work environment. For example, if we are not able to control the temperature or ventilation in our workspace; are impacted by light and noise; don't have easy access to toilets or have to wear synthetic or restrictive workwear.[3] Without support and left to go on for a prolonged period, these symptoms and work conditions can make us feel run down and lead to illness and inability to attend work on some days. We can end up feeling anxious and depressed, and a sense of shame about being menopausal, which leads us to avoid talking about it. In fact, one survey found that of those who needed to take a day off work for menopausal symptoms, 47% reported that they wouldn't tell their employer it was for this reason.[6] So why do so many women find it difficult to talk about menopause at work? Suggested reasons include:

- fear of being seen as weak or incompetent, especially if they work in very competitive environments and have worked hard to get to their position.
- concern about job security; especially if their employer is looking to reduce the workforce, women may feel vulnerable to draw attention to their age or difficulties at work.

- stigma – women can feel embarrassed and unable to disclose their menopausal difficulties and fear they may be stigmatised for being menopausal.[7]

My meno moments

- As with many women, I have had some tough times coping with my symptoms of perimenopause at work. For example, during a week of gushing heavy periods, I was due to give a lecture to around 80 students at a university lecture theatre. I was dreading standing in front of them, but I couldn't cancel last minute as these lectures are booked well in advance and if you don't turn up, you let a lot of people down. I put on lots of extra padding in case of leakage and prepared to travel across London on the underground. I was too scared to sit on the train because of the horrible rush of blood I would feel when I got up, so I stood the whole way. After the hours' journey, I needed to run from the station to the university building, frantically searching for the loo. I entered the lecture theatre feeling flustered, but pleased to see a huge desk and lectern I could stand behind, as cover in case I got a leak. I got through the two-hour lecture and prayed the students wouldn't ask too many questions at the end so I could rush off to the loo again – contrary to the engaging lecturer I like to be!
- There were days when the bleeding was so heavy that I would rush off to the loo every 20 to 30 minutes, hoping no one noticed. And when working in the old NHS hospitals, the toilets were often down a long corridor – making it feel like a walk of shame. Some days I worried I wouldn't be able to drive in without having an 'accident' in the car before I even got into work. I've had to call in sick on one or two days, but 'heavy periods' didn't seem like a plausible reason for sick leave, so I think I said I had 'a bad cold', then worried about whether that makes me look weak to miss work due to a cold.
- Working online from home during Covid lockdowns was a real blessing during those times of heavy unpredictable periods. It could also be helpful in moments of brain fog to quickly google something while on a Zoom call, though of course even that's no good if you can't even think what words to enter in the search tab! And on more than one occasion, I've gone for a tea break or for a walk, relaxed, then suddenly realised about half an hour too late that I was supposed to have joined a work meeting or supervision session.

- When I was going through the worst leg of my perimenopausal journey, I began worrying about my capabilities at work. This was exacerbated by the fact that in the health professions, the concept of 'fitness to practice' is something we are very conscious of in relation to caring for our patients. That's not to say that menopause makes us unfit to practice, but that we can start doubting our abilities in light of the difficulties we are experiencing. If we are not functioning well ourselves, how are we supposed to look after others who are vulnerable and depending on us? Fortunately, I never reached the stage where I was concerned about my ability to provide care and neither did my employers. But my perimenopausal symptoms did make me consider making changes at work, such as cutting down my hours and even contemplate leaving work.
- So, how could I deal with this situation? Should I just throw away all those years of hard work to get to this stage in my career and deprive my clients of the benefit of my skills and experience. Things were eased for me by the fact that I gradually left my NHS job and its constraints to do more independent practice, meaning that I had more autonomy over my work diary and could adapt it to what suited me best. But that is a privilege not afforded to most working women.

Management strategies – for employers and employees

You will have seen in the previous chapters the coping strategies for managing specific symptoms. So, you need to think about how to practicality apply them in your work situation. For example; for hot flushes, it is best to wear removable layers of clothing, avoiding rushing to meetings by planning ahead and being organised; for fatigue, you could make sure you go for a walk at lunch time. On an emotional level, to deal with the unhelpful thoughts and feelings of anxiety and shame that might come up, you can use the 'noticing' and cognitive challenging skills described in Chapters 6 and 7).

In addition to looking after ourselves, what we need from our employers is acknowledgement and support by way of appropriate adjustments so we can continue to function at our best in the workplace and feel supported in looking after our physical and mental health while doing so. The British Standards Institution (BSI) is the UK's official standards body which sets out ways that businesses can improve performance and productivity and look after their employees. It has published a workplace standard for managing 'menstrual and menopausal health matters in your workplace'.[8] Its suggestions, and those in a recent government survey,[3] are incorporated in my list below of strategies that both employers and employees can implement:

Normalising menopause – Employers can encourage more open discussion, for example, by organising workshops and inviting specialist speakers, thus normalising it as a topic. In a more inclusive and supportive environment, women will feel empowered to talk and seek the necessary supports to function at their best. Women can also get together and establish menopause clubs to share experiences to feel supported and less isolated.

Education – Women may have misconceptions around menopause, for example, attributing their symptoms to stress and/or ageing rather than peri- or post-menopause. So, education is needed, not just for them, but also their male, and younger female, colleagues to enable them to understand better and empathise. If there are no such initiatives in your workplace, maybe you can approach your employer to start some.

Training for managers/employers – This is needed for them to understand the potential impact of menopausal symptoms on their staff's functioning at work and how they might provide support. ACAS (the Advisory, Conciliation and Arbitration Service) has been providing such training for a number of years now, covering areas including symptoms, misconceptions, legal considerations and action planning, such as creating a menopause policy.[9]

Work adjustments – Employers should enable and empower women to request adjustments in the workplace that might make things easier for them. For example, line managers could have regular check-ins with employees about their general wellbeing, and if menopause is mentioned, adjustments can be discussed, such as:

- Flexible working – changing working patterns for example, the possibility of having a later start to the day, doing shorter working days, or working from home on some days
- Time allowances – like the option to take more regular breaks, or being given more time to prepare before meetings, appointments or other tasks
- Practical adjustments – like being given a desk fan, being seated at a cooler part of the office or within easy access to the toilets, being permitted to make changes to uniforms so they are more comfortable and so on

You can talk to your line manager in the first instance if you feel comfortable in doing so. Otherwise, you might go to the occupational health service and ask them to help you arrange support and possible work adjustments. Like we discussed in Chapter 9 about tracking your symptoms and making your list before going to see your doctor, you can make a list of how your symptoms make things difficult for you at work and think ahead about the practical changes you'd like to suggest that might help you. Managers will generally appreciate it if you have 'solved the problem' to some extent and they just need to think about how to implement it. Of course, some work situations where you need adjustments may have wider implications in the organisation, so you would also need to give them time to work out a solution.

The organisation, Menopause in the Workplace Limited, in partnership with the University of Warwick, has produced a '5-minute guide: Talking to your manager about menopause' in which the steps are:[10]

- Prepare for your meeting – Check out what policies or support your organisation might already have in place – if there's nothing there, talk to the Human Resources team. Keep a diary of symptoms and ideas about what might help, as mentioned above.
- Book a meeting – So you are given enough time and a private space to talk.
- Explain your situation clearly – Having your notes here will help.
- Let your manager know if you want the conversation to be kept confidential – It's up to you if are happy talking about menopause openly with your colleagues or not.
- Follow up – Agree another meeting time to formalise a way forward, monitor progress or discuss updates as your situation might change.

Emotional and mental health support – Employers should offer counselling or CBT where needed via the employee assist programme if they have one or encourage employees to seek it via their GP. A simple self-help CBT booklet provided as a resource has been shown to be a potentially effective management tool for some women.[11] They could also train up 'menopause champions' to provide informal support.

Creating policies – Women at work need to be given clearly set-out guidelines about what provisions their employer has in place for managing menopause at work and what the procedures are for them to access support.

Addressing inequalities – There are a number of ways women may be unfairly treated due to their menopausal symptoms. For example, they should not be forced to take annual leave to cover days off due to menopausal symptoms, and these absences should be recorded separately to their overall attendance record so as not to unfairly count against them. Difficulties with menopause can potentially lead to further inequalities for minority groups, people with disabilities, and women from Black and ethnic minority backgrounds, so employers need to be aware of and prevent such inequalities.[3]

Legal processes – It is, of course, best if employers and employees communicate well from the start to resolve issues in the workplace to avoid things escalating to the potential for legal action. However, if it comes to it, you should be aware that although there is yet to be specific legislation for menopause at work, issues of complaint against your employer may be covered by the following acts of law:

- Equality Act 2010, which protects workers against discrimination
- Health and Safety at Work Act 1974, which says an employer must, where reasonably practical, ensure everyone's health, safety and welfare at work

Although the menopause is not an illness or disability, the effects of the symptoms experienced can be disabling for women, which means that employers who fail to properly support women could be found to be discriminatory. Precedence has been set by a number of cases where women have taken their employer to court and been awarded damages. For example, Karen Farquharson, an office manager, successfully sued her employer for unfair dismissal and harassment about the time she had to take off sick due to her menopausal symptoms and was awarded £37,000 in damages. Social worker, Maria Rooney, initiated legal action against her employer, Leicester city council in the first case involving an employment tribunal where menopause symptoms are considered a disability for the purposes of the Equality Act and was supported by the Equality and Human Rights Commission (EHRC).

If we don't ask, we won't get!

When I was younger, I never had the confidence to ask for special consideration at work for my cultural/religious needs. It was not an issue of shame as I was always proud to say I am Muslim and talk about my cultural customs. It was probably more about fitting in, not wanting to 'make a fuss'. For example, when I observed my fasting during Ramadan in the winter months the time for breaking my fast would be around 4 p.m., and if I was due to be in a meeting then I would take a bottle of water and a couple of dates in with me, which I quietly consumed when the time came to break my fast. Most people probably didn't even notice. But ideally, I should have excused myself from the meeting at the appropriate time. Then I could have my water, dates and maybe a little snack, found a space to say my obligatory prayers and then gone back to the meeting. I have the confidence to do this now, well more so than before.

Likewise, I suppose I didn't want to ask for special consideration for my peri-menopausal physical needs. Apart from 'not making a fuss', I think this probably did involve an element of shame. It would draw attention to my ageing, and it seemed too personal and too 'messy' to talk about. The latter was probably related to my upbringing in thinking of 'women's issues' as taboo topics.

When I started reading about the issues related to menopause and work, it made me think of how things were in relation to mental health issues and work. And more specifically for women, if we go back further in employment law, it is also probably similar to the struggles related to pregnancy at work and maternity leave. It may be that not all workplaces will encourage or willingly entertain the idea of making allowances for menopausal experiences, but seeing the recent interest in menopause as a topic in the media generally, including in political campaigning, there is hope that workplaces will adapt, and the necessary legislation and policies will follow.

Reviewing support in the workplace, a recent UK government survey found that:[3]

- Just under 11% of respondents requested adjustments due to their symptoms – the most common requests were for flexible working and temperature control.
- Of those who did not request adjustments, the main reason given was 'I was worried about the reaction of others' (26%) and 'I didn't know who to speak to' (19%).
- The majority of those who requested an adjustment received some form of adjustment; however, 30% received no adjustments. Of those who received adjustment, 55% found those adjustments helpful.

So, clearly, employers have some way to go in supporting women going through the menopause in the workplace. And we also need to continue to speak up about menopause and develop the confidence to ask for what we need and want. One positive move is that the UK government has pledged to 'open up the conversation, tackle stigma and be aware of the menopause – particularly how it affects individuals in their career and the workplace'. A Menopause Employment Champion has been appointed as an ambassador to drive forward this agenda.[12]

In summary, it is increasingly being recognised that the menopausal transition can have significant impacts on women during their working lives. Employers need to recognise this and women need to be empowered to talk about it and request appropriate adjustments, rather than 'hide' their symptoms, suffer in silence or leave their jobs (where they can) when it gets too much. By giving proper attention to menopause and treating it as an occupational health concern and providing reasonable adjustments as required, employers can ensure that women are motivated and productive to their full capacity and less likely to need days off sick, hold back on their careers, or even leave work, taking all that talent and experience with them.

Key points

Remember you are not alone with menopause at work

Don't be afraid to ask for any adjustments you need

Employers have started to take notice of the menopause and its impact

Today I am grateful for:

The opportunity of education and a long career I still enjoy

Good colleagues and considerate managers

The flexibility I've been lucky to take advantage of in my work life

Your turn:

List your **key learning points** from this chapter

List two or three things (big or small) you are **grateful for** right now

16 Cultural Differences in Experience, Attitude and Coping

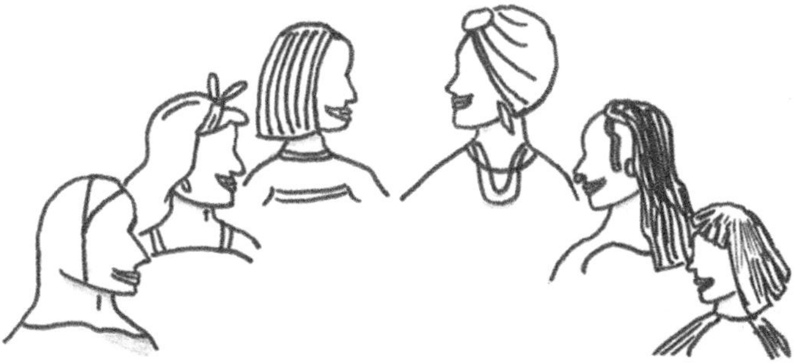

As we have seen so far, we all have our individual experiences of the journey from perimenopause through menopause and into postmenopause. But what about the social contexts in which we experience this transition – does that play a part? Straddling two cultures, I am curious about variations in experiences. So, I wondered if there were any actual differences in the way we experience menopause based on our race or ethnicity, and if so, what might the underlying contributory factors be? And are there any significant differences in the way we manage our symptoms based on our cultural backgrounds?

Much of the reporting on racial and ethnic differences in women's experience of the menopause transition and health during mid-life comes from the Study of Women's Health Across the Nation (SWAN).[1] This is the largest longitudinal study in this field, which started in 1996 and is ongoing today. The researchers enrolled 3,302 women who were then aged between 42 and 52 years old. They came from a number of cities across USA, from a range of socioeconomic backgrounds, and from the following five racial/ethnic groups: White (46%); African American (28%); Hispanic (9%), Chinese (8%) and Japanese (9%). The researchers have been studying the physical, biological, psychological and social changes experienced by these women during this transitional period and have produced well over 600 published papers to date. They have demonstrated some significant racial/ethnic differences in women's experience of the changes during this phase of their lives.

But the SWAN study has its limitations. For example, many ethnic groups are not included. The most glaringly obvious omission to me is that there is no representation of South Asian women like me. There have also been other studies around the world looking into cultural differences, but the sample sizes are often quite small. So, we are in need of more research and representation of all ethnic groups.

Why do we need to study differences?

As most of the research on menopause has historically been done in Western countries, studying mainly White women, it is the experience of these women that has set the context for the way menopause is addressed in healthcare settings. But, as I will discuss below, from the comparatively little research so far in women from other backgrounds, there is quite a diversity in experience. As we don't yet understand much about the nuances in these differences, there are many women left not adequately catered for. This has been known for years now, but even today we are seeing that little advancement has been made in this area. In the UK, a very recent survey of primary care practitioners concluded that: There is a need for increased awareness and trustworthy information resources to help women from ethnic minorities prepare for the menopause and clinicians to recognise their experiences and offer support. This could improve women's immediate quality of life and potentially reduce future disease risk.[2]

Brief summary of differences observed

Here are a few basic findings from research so far:

- White women (European and American) – The average age to reach menopause for women in Western countries is 51 years. White women reported the most sleep complaints and more cognitive symptoms (at more severe levels) than other racial/ethnic groups during their perimenopausal status.[3]
- South Asian women – The average age of menopause in Indian women (living in India) is 46.7 years.[4] Indian women may complain more of vulval and urogynaecological symptoms.[5] The mean age of menopause for Pakistani women is 47.16 years, and significant symptoms reported are headaches, tiredness and joint pain.[6] A recent study in Bangladesh found that the age of menopause varied slightly across regions within the country with the average being 46.7 years.[7] Another study of Bangladeshi women suggests that vasomotor symptoms are more common than previously thought, and joint pain was also commonly reported though it's

suggested this might be linked to physical work as the women studied were fieldworkers.[8]

- Women of African and Caribbean descent – The mean age of menopause for Black women (mostly in American samples) is 49.6 years. Black women experience more vasomotor symptoms than White women, and they tend to be more bothered by them. Also, these symptoms go on for longer, with an average duration of 10 years compared to 6.5 years for White women.[9]
- South-east Asian women – For women of Japanese and Chinese descent, the average age for reaching menopause is 49 years.[10,1] Japanese women report much less experience of vasomotor symptoms – for them, feeling chills and shoulder pain is more common. Chinese and Japanese women may suffer more from forgetfulness, joint and muscle pains.[1]

Some explanations for differences

On some levels, it may be extremely difficult to tease out exactly what factors cause the differences in experience of symptoms and their severity across race, ethnicity and culture. Suggestions of biological, environmental, social and cultural explanations have been put forward to try to make sense of them.

One biological explanation for the differences is the variation in levels of 'oestrogenic activity'. Although we commonly refer to oestrogen as if it were a single hormone, there are actually three subtypes of it – oestrone, oestradiol and oestriol. The combination of these subtypes and their changing levels is referred to as oestrogenic activity. It has been shown that oestrogenic activity is affected by race/ethnicity and can have an impact on menopausal symptoms and average age to reach menopause.[11,12]

There have been two explanations proposed for the difference in the experience of vasomotor symptoms between Western women and Japanese women for example. One suggestion is that because Western women's diets are higher in processed ('damaged') fats and lower in fibre, they accumulate higher levels of oestrogen, so there is a sharper drop in their oestrogen when they hit perimenopause – resulting in a more significant experience of vasomotor symptoms. The other suggestion is that the high intake of phytoestrogens and isoflavones in the Japanese diet lessens the hormonal imbalance they experience.

A suggested explanation for why women of African and Caribbean origin may experience more severe menopausal symptoms and a longer menopause transition than their White counterparts is the potential extra burden placed on their bodies from repeated activation of the stress response due to long-standing gender and racial discrimination and socioeconomic factors.[13]

How culture may influence how we view and experience menopause

I think it is generally accepted that menopause is not thought of in a positive way in Western societies. So, I wondered whether the way we view ageing, women and menopause can make a difference to how we cope with it.

Attitudes towards ageing

There is not a great deal of research into cultural differences in attitudes towards ageing. It is widely believed that Western societies tend to have a more youth-focused attitude, and so place more value in young adults over older adults. Conversely, Eastern societies are generally considered to be more accepting of older adults and teaching the younger generation to respect, obey and care for their elders.

One study aimed to test the idea that Eastern cultures hold older people in higher regard than Western cultures by collecting data from 507 university students in the UK and Taiwan.[14] They examined concepts such as cultural norms about older people and the students' personal attitudes. They actually found that it was not as clear-cut as we might think. There were some aspects in which both the UK and Taiwanese students had relatively positive personal attitudes towards older people. And they also identified among the Taiwanese students that there were some aspects about older people they considered positively and other aspects they considered negatively. This pointed to the idea of a co-existence of both positive and negative views about older people in the East. These findings suggest that perhaps we shouldn't generalise so readily about cultural biases towards ageing and more research is required. This study did not differentiate between attitudes towards older men and older women, and I think this would be another interesting area to explore – are the East and/or West more ageist towards women than men?

I also wonder whether attitudes towards ageing have changed over time, perhaps in all cultures. Growing up in my Bangladeshi community, I noticed that my parents, uncles and aunts looked forward to getting older. I think that was because being the 'senior' in the family was a position of respect and honour. It was a patriarchal society like most, of course, but even for women, if you were older, you were still granted this status. I would see grown men still being told what to do by their mothers and not confronting them. My own paternal grandmother was a forceful character, and I recall my father's frustrations at times when he would consult her (she was the head of the household since my grandfather had passed away) about important family matters and she'd make decisions he disagreed with. He couldn't not consult her, nor defy her outright, because he needed her blessing. Now, in a modern Western society that might be seen as a man being emasculated, but of course, they could negotiate on important matters. My point is that the elders held a status of high esteem – they were not invisible little old people tucked away in some corner, but sat in a position of power. Having recently visited Bangladesh, I observed respect for the elders is still fairly strong – perhaps more so in rural communities than in urban ones. However, I suspect things are changing in Asian families living in the West. I know my mother gets upset sometimes when my siblings and I make decisions about family matters and 'forget' to consult her.

Attitudes towards fertility and ageing in women

Perhaps in all societies, a woman is most visible in her earlier, fertile years. As she ages, she is viewed as losing her attractiveness. You'll know by now that I'm into films. I recall a scene in a Lebanese film called Caramel (2007) – when an older woman, Jamale, goes for an acting audition and applies fake blood on the back of her skirt so others will assume she is still menstruating and had a 'leak', hence still fertile, desirable and castable in a film. It made me sad that she should feel so ashamed of her ageing and loss of fertility, and that scene has stuck in my mind since watching it about 15 years ago. This shame about no longer being feminine and fertile is a reflection of the fact that in many societies, being postmenopausal somehow renders you as no longer serving a purpose. 'You're no longer attractive *and* you can't bear children, so step aside please' seems to be the message. Fortunately, this is not the case in all societies, as we'll go on to see.

Biologists and anthropologists have come up with a scientific explanation as to why we are one of the few species who live beyond our fertile years and tried to give an evolutionary purpose to menopause by suggesting that it plays an adaptive role in the survival of the gene pool. This 'grandmother hypothesis'[15] suggests that as women age, there is more advantage in older women putting their energies into helping their existing offsprings in their reproductive efforts rather than having more children of their own. That is, postmenopausal women have a role in contributing to bringing up the next generation.

Although there are one or two criticisms of the grandmother hypothesis, it is a helpful way of looking at the purposeful role older women can play. I know I, for one, needed my mother to look after my first child when I went back to work after maternity leave. Yes, there were nurseries, which I did use later, but when your child is very young, it can be more reassuring to leave them in the trusting and doting arms of your mother, where this is possible of course. There are many women who rely on their mothers to help, and given the cost of paid childcare these days, it makes economic sense for many families. It is often a mutually rewarding experience of quality time between the grandmother and the grandchild. I believe spending my early years in an intergenerational household gave me a rich bonding experience, which I appreciate.

The grandmother role is also about giving advice, not just on child-rearing but life in general – and not necessarily just within their own family. One excellent idea for tapping into grandmothers as a source of support is the Friendship Bench project developed by psychiatrist Dr Chibanda in Zimbabwe. This project trains grandmothers to deliver an evidence-based problem-solving therapy to those in their community who are suffering from common mental health disorders, such as anxiety and depression, and has been found to be effective.[16]

Attitudes towards menopause and the influence on experience

Numerous studies have demonstrated that our experience of menopausal symptoms is strongly influenced by the cultural environment in which we live.[17] Whereas in the West, we define menopause as the *ending* of something (menstrual cycles and fertility), in China, it is seen as the *start* of a new phase of life, a 'rebirth'; a time when energy that was used for reproductive purposes can be saved. In Japan too, it is seen as a time to start anew. The Japanese word for menopause is *konenki*, which could be translated into 'years/season of renewal/regeneration'. Perhaps this positive framing of menopause correlates with Chinese and Japanese women reportedly having an easier time of it. A positive mindset leading to a more positive experience. The Japanese have only recently created an equivalent phrase for the English phrase 'hot flush' – 'hotto furasshu' – as none existed before. It will be interesting to see in future research if the incidence of hot flushes increases among Japanese women now that they have a word for it.

Mayan women in Mexico and Central America typically experience menopause up to 10 years earlier than their U.S. counterparts. However, their symptoms have a shorter duration, they don't generally use HRT and appear to have a lower prevalence of osteoporosis. Apart from genetics and a predominately plant-based diet, it is thought that their attitude plays a significant part in experiencing an easier menopause transition. There is also no stigma associated with ageing and menopause within their culture, giving them a more positive outlook. Postmenopausal Mayan women also acquire a new status of becoming spiritual leaders of their communities, especially those in the more rural regions.[18]

In India, there is a cultural view that menstruation is polluting, which means that when they are on their period, women are restricted from entering places that are considered sacred or pure.[19] But, this can put a positive twist on menopause, because when they are postmenopausal and no longer having periods, these restrictions are lifted and they are free to join in more cultural events. This is also generally the case for Muslim women in Asia and the Middle East. In one study of Arabic women, although the term for menopause ('the hopeless age') has negative connotations, many women reported being more socially active in postmenopause. They could now take part in religious activities that were previously off limits while they were menstruating and see this phase as a time of renewed life, greater inclusion, and higher position in society.[20]

It's also important to look at differences *within* the larger ethnic groups rather than treating them as a homogenous group. A closer look at American Asians found that Filipino Americans reported more positive attitudes towards menopause and milder symptoms than Chinese and Korean Americans.[21] Even across European countries, differences in experience and attitude have been observed – the European Menopause Survey revealed that women in the UK had more severe symptoms compared to those in Spain and France.[22] In Sweden, Denmark and Norway, where there is a positive view of ageing and menopause, women reported experiencing fewer symptoms and said it was better than they had expected.[23]

It may be said that in some cultures, women are not encouraged to express their discomfort with menopausal symptoms. For example, it is suggested that perhaps Indian women do not report their menopausal symptoms, because they attribute them to ageing rather than menopause or because talking about menstruation and menopause is still taboo in Indian culture and presumably South Asian cultures in general.[19] But, there are indications that things are starting to change, at least in more urban societies perhaps, as shown for example by a recent article in the Times of India newspaper with the headline 'The "ladies problem" that is no longer a taboo topic'.[24] It describes women who are 'tapping into [their] sisterhood' by, for example, creating a paid membership support group. It also mentions a health platform and app, which reports that more than 55,000 women have enrolled on its menopause management programmes.

In summary, women from cultures that perceive menopause positively generally experience fewer and less bothersome symptoms than women from cultures that associate menopause with ageing and view ageing in a negative light.[23] Similarly, a review investigating the relationship between attitude and experience found that in 10 out of the 13 studies, women with more negative attitudes towards the menopause report more symptoms.[25]

What about those not living in their country of origin?

So, what about women like me who were born in one country but grew up in, or moved to, another country – what should they expect? Is our experience likely to be more akin to those from the country and culture of our origin or those living in the same cultural environment? It looks like this is a complex question and will depend on many factors including the degree of acculturation – the extent to which you maintain the primary aspects of your identity while integrating aspects of the culture of the society in which you currently live. Having lived in the UK since childhood, I most often identify with the attitudes of British culture, but I am also mindful of the influences of my culture of origin. I wonder what this means for my menopause experience, at least the aspects not influenced by genetics.

One Australian study reported that 'cultural conditioning' plays a significant role in the reporting of menopausal symptoms. They found that Chinese women living in Sydney had a slightly higher prevalence of vasomotor symptoms than Chinese women in Mainland China or Hong Kong, but a lower prevalence of symptoms than White women.[26] And the level of symptom reporting was higher among women who had lived in Australia for 10 years or more.

A UK-based study collected data on lifestyle, general health, menopause experience and help-seeking behaviour of three groups of peri- and postmenopausal women aged 45–55 years: 52 Asian women originating from the Indian subcontinent living in Birmingham, UK; 51 White women living in the same geographical area; 50 Asian women living in Delhi, India. They found that the UK Asian women's experience of the menopause is more similar to the White women in the UK than that of the women in Delhi.[27]

Another study which aimed to investigate the potential influence of acculturation, compared 17 studies on Asian women living in Asia and those living in Western countries. They found that Asian women in Western societies were not highly acculturated and retained traditional practices. Their religion and cultural influences promoted a sense of acceptance and neutrality about menopause. However, they also held conflicted views on whether menopause represented the loss of femininity and youthfulness or the beginning of a new life.[25]

Are there inequalities in menopause care based on ethnicity?

Studies have shown that there are potential racial biases at play in the care for menopausal symptoms for women of Black and ethnic minority backgrounds, whether in the UK or USA.[28] For example, a 2023 UK study revealed that doctors with the highest proportion of patients from ethnic minorities spent far less on HRT than those with the highest proportion of White patients, so White women were significantly more likely to be prescribed HRT.[29] A survey of primary care practitioners in the UK reported that in recent years they had seen a marked increase in the number of women seeking support for menopausal symptoms, which they mainly attributed to more media campaigns. However, this did not include women from ethnic minority groups in the population – they were not coming forth any more than they did before. Why was that? Were they not experiencing the same degree of symptoms? Or, was it more likely that the campaigning did not speak to them – the images used in the media posters did not represent them?[2]

For Asian women, in addition to not being adequately catered for in campaigns, the conservative nature of their cultures may be a factor – making them hesitate to speak about what are seen as intimate health issues – creating a barrier to accessing timely and appropriate treatment. And when asked, Asian women mentioned the need for family support and understanding of what they were experiencing. So, there is a need for culturally sensitive educational resources for menopausal women and their family members to increase awareness and appropriate knowledge and to promote communication about menopause.[25]

Given the impact that menopause can have on the quality of women's lives, inequalities can have a big impact on their health and wellbeing. All women need to be educated not only on the symptoms of perimenopause and postmenopause and how to seek help for this, but also about other related risks. For example, the younger you are when you start menopause, the higher your risk of cardiovascular disease and death – so you would need more advice on looking after your heart. The British Menopause Society highlights the need for further research and states that 'the influence of culture, race and ethnicity on attitudes towards menopausal symptoms and treatment is very complex ... The menopause transition in ethnic minority women remains poorly understood, with a big gap in service provision'.[30]

Cultural difference in coping approaches

East meets West – and mother knows best ...

Growing up in the UK, I became more inclined towards the conventional Western approaches to health and medicine than the practices of my Eastern heritage. I reacted with teenage disdain at my mother's 'alternative' suggestions for managing our health and wellbeing – for example, when we were slightly under the weather, she was more likely to slice up some ginger to chew or put in a soothing tea or use turmeric to make a milky concoction before reaching for a bottle of cough or cold medicine. I often rolled my eyes at her use of oils. And don't get me started on our battles over putting coconut oil in my hair! But now, I have a stock of oil products in my kitchen cupboard and buy ginger shots and turmeric lattes at high street cafes, as my Western world has cottoned on to the benefits of such ingredients. I'm ashamed to admit I thought my mother was 'backward' for using charcoal powder (bought from a Bangladeshi shop here or sent over by relatives) for whitening her teeth. But guess what I've been using from time to time to get whiter teeth? That's right, a pricey, nicely packaged charcoal toothpaste. Don't tell Mum!

My mother would use these strategies, because they were handed down to her and it was what she knew and trusted. But she was not aware of the 'science' behind these practices, and she got frustrated when asked to explain. As I've grown older and being naturally avoidant of medication (or rather I expect there was some maternal influence there), I've been more open to exploring the Eastern perspective on healthcare. Being more educated, I was able to research and evaluate how they work and make informed choices about them. I then realised that not everything my mother suggested was a 'crack-pot' idea or an 'old wives' tale. And there is something about my mother's faith in what her ancestors passed down that I have come to appreciate too.

So, now while exploring ways of coping with menopause, I'm wondering whether there might be ways of coping with the symptoms that we in the West haven't thought of and which might make it into our mainstream practice, as indeed practices like mindfulness and meditation already have. But I have found that the research in this area is scant. We know there are differences in experiences and attitudes, and we have learnt about dietary differences and lifestyle playing a part, but there seems to be little exploration of whether women in different societies tackle their specific symptoms differently and what their practices might be. So again, more research is needed.

Differences in approach to management of symptoms

In summarising the findings from SWAN and a couple of other longitudinal studies in the USA, one review paper reported the following differences among ethnic groups:[31]

- *Seeking information or advice* – Most White women visited their doctors for care and advice to manage their menopausal symptoms. It was thought that they predominately viewed menopausal symptoms as a serious health issue that they would have to endure for a long time. On the contrary, many ethnic minority women turned to their elders first, then close friends as their main source of information and advice. Asian women predominately believed that menopause is part of the normal ageing process and tended not to seek care.
- *Medication as the first or final choice* – While White women preferred to take a variety of different medications to alleviate their symptoms and turned to medication first, ethnic minority women commonly tended to use medication as a last resort when alternative approaches had failed.
- *Treating specific symptoms or holistic approach* – White women largely preferred symptom-focused management strategies or treatments, whereas

ethnic minority women preferred holistic 'mind–body–spirit' strategies to relieve menopausal symptoms and feel better as a whole.

- *Approach to diet* – White women tended to use the approach of avoiding certain 'trigger' foods, whereas ethnic minority women actively pursued health foods to improve their general health.
- *Complementary or Alternative Treatment (CAM)* Although it was found that there was significant use of CAM across all ethnic groups, there were still differences observed. White and Japanese women had the highest rates of use (60%) followed by Chinese women (46%), African American (40%) and Hispanic (20%) women. All groups stopped using CAM once they reached menopause.

In conclusion on cultural differences

In summary, studies have for some time shown that our ethnicity can actually influence our peri- and post-menopausal experiences and even *when* we reach menopause. Although it is generally thought that environmental factors, such as lifestyle and socioeconomic status, are probably mostly accountable for these racial/ethnic differences, variations in our experiences of the menopause may be attributed to our cultural perceptions which shape our expectations. There are societies in which menopause is equated with old age and ageing is dreaded, leading to a negative view of menopause as it is seen as a time of loss – loss of youth, physical and sexual attractiveness and fertility. In other societies, there is generally a greater acceptance of ageing and it is equated to wisdom. Here, despite the loss of fertility, postmenopausal women embrace it with a positive mindset, as a time of gain – in terms of rejuvenation, newfound freedom and improved social status, which presumably gives them greater self-esteem. Perhaps this should give us some food for thought in the West about how we educate and campaign to reduce the stigma associated with ageing and menopause to promote a more positive attitude.

Let me give you a little exercise here: Have a think about your own attitudes around ageing and menopause? Where might they stem from? To what extent are they cultural or societal or individual thoughts? And more importantly, do you think your attitudes might be helping or hindering you own experience of menopause?

Studies, such as SWAN, provide a good foundation for understanding racial, ethnic and cultural differences in the menopause experience. However, on the whole, there is still a large gap in knowledge in this field. More research is needed to better understand the differences and the variations in perceptions, attitudes and expectations around menopause. Increasing our understanding may lead to healthcare providers offering more fitting care and the promotion of lifestyles that may improve the management of, or experience of symptoms, and increase quality of life for all women.

Key points

Culture influences experience, attitudes and approaches to coping with symptoms.

More research is needed on differences in experiences

Inequalities need to be addressed and more culturally-nuanced care provided

Today I am grateful for:

My ancestral line of strong matriarchs

Both the Eastern and Western influences in my life experience

Being in a position to pick the best from both, and open-minded about potential solutions

Your turn:

List your **key learning points** from this chapter

List two or three things (big or small) you are **grateful for** right now

Part IV

Conclusion

17 The Onward Journey

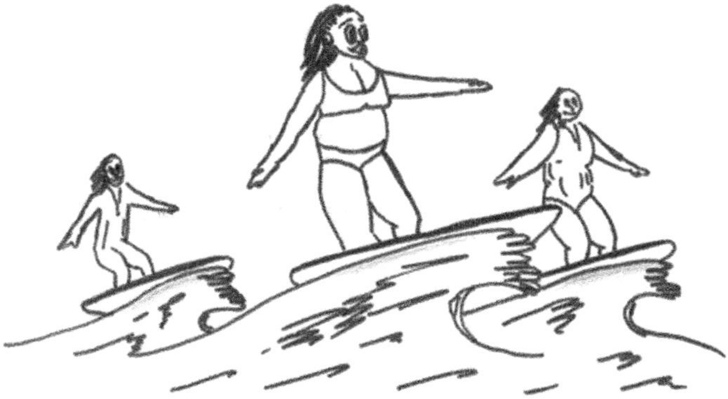

Although menopause can be a fairly straight-forward transition for some women, maybe even hardly noticed, for many of us, it can cause quite a ripple and turn into a long-drawn-out and tiresome journey. For others still it can be a devastating time, even leading to thoughts of suicide. Wherever, our experience lies on this continuum, there are ways to manage and reduce our distress. It is no longer acceptable to suffer in silence or become invisible to the world.

Stigma has historically surrounded menopause and ageing in women generally. This has meant that women's issues in middle age and beyond, such as menopause, have not gained much traction', with regard to advancements in approaches to the management of symptoms. Challenging this gendered ageism is quite a task, but it is being taken on by more and more researchers and campaigners in the field (see Resources). I see it as a challenge both within and outside of ourselves. On an internal level for example, how do we view our own ageing process and menopause? As we have seen, social and cultural factors play a significant part in our attitude towards, expectations of, and experiences of menopause. Women who perceive menopause positively generally experience fewer and less bothersome symptoms than those who associate menopause with ageing and view ageing in a negative light. Perhaps we can take a leaf out of the books of our sisters in other parts of the world, like China and Japan, and see it as a new beginning or second spring, rather than an ending, or a time of demise.

I care about my appearance and youthfulness as much as the next woman. But it is a strange dichotomy to be part of an environment with a positive attitude towards ageing, while at the same time often hearing the words, 'what will people think?". The poem 'Warning' by Jenny Joseph struck a chord with me even in my teenage years. It speaks of old age as a time of increased freedom when one no longer needs to conform to the conventional rules of society. I sometimes quote the line, 'When I am an old woman, I shall wear purple' as a sort of mantra. The Bangladeshi in me has no qualms about wearing purple and red together, as Jenny suggests. Bangladeshis are a fairly non-conformist bunch by nature, but I can't say I've had the courage to go the whole hog to 'make up for the sobriety of my youth'. I do think it's time I start practising though. What's the point of going through the aches of menopause if I don't throw caution to the wind now? As a result, I think I'm ready to embrace the 'auntie' role. There's a joke among Bangladeshis about how our elders tend to speak in rhymes – for example, 'Do you want some biscuit-tiscuit with your tea?'. With that in mind and my new-found menopausal freedom, I say '"ageing bageing, bring it on!"'

On an external level of course, we need society to shift too. And here, education is key. That's education for everyone, not just us as women. Menopause is not just about us – the half of the population going through it – it concerns everyone. As we have seen, what we go through has an impact not just on our lives, but also those around us and the wider society. So, we all need to be in this together – all being educated about it. Children need to be taught about it at school, doctors and therapists need more specialist training, employers need to understand how they can help and policy-makers need to keep it on their agenda. It's reassuring to see that there are positive movements in all these areas. If we look at how far we have come with discussing mental health issues, I believe the stigma towards menopause and ageing in women is also slowly shifting. But it will take time.

Menopause is a time of significant change, and although that can be a difficult process for many, with knowledge, resources and support, it does not have to be – nor indeed should it be – a miserable journey. As it is a natural part of life that all women will experience, we don't want to pathologise it, that is, treat it like something psychologically abnormal. And neither should we medicalise it, that is, we should not view it as a medical condition that necessitates hormonal or medical treatment. We need a 'realistic and balanced' narrative around the management of menopause.[1] Given the neglect in this area for so long, researchers also need to keep investigating the experience of menopause and finding more solutions for managing the symptoms – medical or otherwise. I recommend keeping an open mind about what we can learn from different cultures as a way of tapping into as yet unconsidered solutions that could potentially be proven to work effectively.

It is important to normalise menopause so that women feel able to speak about it openly and get the support they need in all areas of their lives. In today's society, social media and celebrity are often the way we tend to measure what's popular and what then becomes 'normal' to talk about. Women from many fields have shared their menopausal experiences publicly in recent years including, Davina McCall, Emma Thompson, Gabby Logan, Shania Twain and Michelle Obama, to name just a few. I don't think it's simply my selective attention to the topic or the algorithms at play, but there is generally more chatter about menopause on social media and I have recently seen more mention of menopause in the mainstream media. Though we should also be cautious about misinformation and unscrupulous marketing, as the menopausal woman is currently a target for all kinds of new manipulative sales opportunities.

Going by the number of books coming out on menopause, the online groups available to join and the access of in-person meet-ups like 'menopause cafes' (see Resources), it seems there is a thirst for knowledge and a desire to come together to talk about it. I have mentioned how sharing our experiences helps us feel less isolated and can give us access to sources of support. Knowledge leads to empowerment. Just knowing what is going on with our bodies and minds during this time is a relief in itself. Having access to strategies, tools and treatments gives us confidence that we can navigate menopause. We should celebrate all that we have gained in our years so far – experience, knowledge, wisdom and courage, to name but a few attributes. This time of change can be reframed as a time of growth for us and a time for society to embrace us in our middle age and senior years. Far from being invisible, we should be seen as a useful resource to tap into. All in all, I am hopeful that the forecast is good for society to acknowledge the impact of menopause on women and make shifts towards accommodating it and integrating it into everyday life.

In talking of education, I'm reminded that at school we are taught that a story should have a beginning, middle and end. Well, I was at primary school when my menstrual story started, and though the beginning of my perimenopausal journey was hard to track, it has pretty much covered a lot of my middle age so far. As I write, I am still not quite at the 'end' – I'm still eagerly waiting to transition from the perimenopausal leg of this journey to hit that moment clinically defined as 'menopause'. I have again gone six months without bleeding, so who knows I could make it to twelve. Or I might have to hit the re-set button any time now. I've heard many women talk about looking forward to and celebrating that moment, as I have done myself. And I've heard others question, 'What's the point when you can still be experiencing symptoms in postmenopause?'. So, while for some, it might just be an arbitrary moment in time, for others it's a rite of passage into the next phase, even if that phase might not look too different form the previous one for some years. The ending of periods may be seen as a welcome and freeing experience for some women, but perhaps a loss of womanhood for others. It's about perspective.

One of the things I hope I've shown in this book is how our perspective and attitudes make a difference to how we cope with menopause. So, rather than seeing it as the 'beginning of the end', as my cousin put it, I can acknowledge that while, at times it has been a somewhat turbulent journey, during which I've hit a few storms, the clouds are now clearing. I am still experiencing a few symptoms but on the whole, I am feeling immensely better than I did before I started writing this book. In fact, when I read back on my descriptions of my symptoms, I now don't even remember how some of them felt. So, I'm glad I chose to write about them as I was experiencing them. It may be that my symptoms are naturally easing off, as they do for many women, but I also believe it's because I have better knowledge about how my body works and how to use my coping strategies effectively. I am now riding the waves rather than frantically battling against them, feeling out of my depth and buffeted about. If you recall the quicksand metaphor in Chapter 8, there is similar advice for survival in dangerous water – don't fight the water but try to float on it, maintain your energy levels and be more visible to those trying to rescue you. In the choppy waters of menopause, there is a lot you can do to rescue yourself. The support and help of friends and professionals can make it easier too – so don't be afraid to seek this out.

If you are yet to start on this journey, I hope you feel well informed with my personal experiences and insights on what the symptoms can look and feel like. If you are currently experiencing peri- or postmenopausal symptoms, I hope they don't feel too overwhelming, and more so, that you now feel better equipped and confident about managing your symptoms using the holistic approach I have put forward. At this stage in your life, you are likely to have many demands on your time. Of course, you can't make your personal and professional responsibilities just disappear, but I hope I have encouraged you to reflect a little on your priorities and to make even some small changes that could make life run more smoothly. Let menopause be a time when you are kind to yourself, turn up for yourself, give value to your own time and feel empowered to spend it as you wish, doing what is meaningful to you and brings you joy. This will have a positive impact not only on your menopause experience, but also your overall sense of wellbeing and in turn how you relate to others. That can only be a good thing for everyone!

I wish you all the best on your onward journey.

Key points

You are now armed with the knowledge, tools and strategies to enjoy a healthy and smooth menopausal journey.

You are now empowered – ask for what you need at the doctors, at work and at home!

Be kind to yourself and enjoy life!

Today I am grateful for:

Finishing writing this book – it's been a rewarding experience

All the good people in my life – friends, family and supporters

My faith – the peace, comfort and sense of contentment it gives me

Your turn:

List your **key learning points** from this book

List two or three things (big or small) you are **grateful for** right now

Further Support and Resources

Mental health concerns

As we have seen, the myriad of potential symptoms can make navigating menopause quite difficult. It is essential to have reliable sources of information and support. In Chapter 5, I discussed that although menopause is a biological process during which time many physical symptoms are encountered, it can often create emotional turmoil and lead to challenging psychological symptoms. Some women may find that menopause leads to or exacerbates mental health difficulties, such as anxiety disorders or depression. You might experience a number of the symptoms below during some part of your menopausal transition.

Symptoms of depression:

- Feeling down or hopeless
- Little interest or pleasure in things you usually enjoy
- Feeling bad about yourself
- Feeling irritable
- Feeling tired, lacking energy
- Difficulty concentrating
- Difficulty sleeping or wanting to sleep all the time
- Loss of appetite or overeating
- Thoughts of suicide or of not wanting to be around

Symptoms of anxiety:

- Feeling nervous or anxious
- Difficulty relaxing
- Ongoing worrying thoughts
- Worrying about lots of different things
- Fearing the worst
- Feeling irritable
- Feeling restless or agitated

If you find you are experiencing several of these symptoms persistently, you should reach out for further help. Please don't feel you have to cope on your own. There is help available. It is also important that you let a family member or friend know how you're feeling so that they can help you to access the support you need and hopefully be available as an additional source of support.

Where to seek further support

1. Your GP is your first port of call for discussing mental health difficulties as well as physical health problems. They will know what general mental health support is available in your area. Although you may find it difficult to approach your GP about your mental health, especially if you don't see the same one regularly, it is really important that you do share your concerns about your mental health difficulties with them, so they can refer you to the most appropriate service.
2. Your GP may refer you to your local Talking Therapies Service (previously known as Improving Access to Psychological Therapies or IAPT). Alternatively, you should be able to refer yourself by contacting them directly. These services offer short-term counselling and therapies for people experiencing common mental health difficulties. More information can be found on the NHS website.
3. If you wish to see a psychologist privately, it is important to ensure you see someone who is highly trained and regulated. The term 'psychologist' is not currently a protected title in the UK. Therefore, you should seek someone who is registered with the Health and Care Professions Council (HCPC). Anyone calling themselves a clinical, health or counselling psychologist should be registered with HCPC. You can check the register on the HCPC website. For more on finding a clinical psychologist, the Association of Clinical Psychologists UK (ACP-UK) has a useful guide on its website.
4. Connecting with other women going through menopause can provide valuable insights and emotional support. You might look out for support groups in your area, such as a Menopause Café (see Further reading and resources below).

If you are at risk to yourself

Again, as discussed in Chapter 2, for some women, their symptoms may be so severe and debilitating that they will contemplate ending their life. They might have fleeting suicidal thoughts or the thoughts might become more frequent and concerning. As stated above, thoughts of suicide or not wanting to be around can be an indication of depression. If you notice *any of the* symptoms below, then you should seek immediate help:

- Being preoccupied with thoughts of death or dying
- Making a plan of how you would end your life
- Taking steps to say goodbye to loved ones
- Acquiring things to follow through your plan
- Writing a suicide note

Where to seek further crisis support

1. It is important to let your GP know about any of these symptoms. Ask for an urgent appointment.
2. If you live in England, you can access the NHS Urgent Mental Health helpline via the NHS website. There is also a mental health text support service which you can access by texting SHOUT to 85258.
3. The Samaritans are trained to support people who are feeling suicidal. You can call them for free at any time on 116 123. Or check their website for other ways to get in touch with them.
4. If you are concerned that you are at high or immediate risk of suicide, then you should go to the Accident and Emergency Department at your local hospital. There will be a psychiatric liaison team on duty who can assess you and work with you to develop an immediate plan to support you.

Further reading and resources

Here are some books and resources that you might find helpful for understanding and managing your symptoms:

Espie, Colin (2021) *Overcoming Insomnia 2nd Edition: A self-help guide using cognitive behavioural techniques.* Overcoming Books Series.

Gurney, Karen (2020) *Mind the Gap: The Truth About Desire and How to Futureproof Your Sex Life.* Headline Publishing Group Ltd.

Meadows, Guy (2014) *The Sleep Book: How to Sleep Well Every Night.* Orion Publishing Group.

Mosconi, Lisa (2020) *THE XX BRAIN: The Groundbreaking Science Empowering Women to Maximize Cognitive Health and Prevent Alzheimer's Disease.* Allen & Unwin.

National Autistic Society (2024) *Autism and Menopause.* https://www.autism.org.uk

Sim, Stacy (2022) *Next Level: Your Guide to Kicking Ass, Feeling Great, and Crushing Goals Through Menopause and Beyond.* Rodale Books.

International Menopause Society – videos and podcasts of interviews with the world's leading experts on different topics related to menopause: https://www.menopauseinfo.org/videos/

Further information about diet from The British Dietetic Association: https://www.bda.uk.com/

MakeMenopauseMatter campaign: https://menopausesupport.co.uk/

Menopause Research and Education Fund: https://mref.uk/mref-resources/

Menopause clinics/specialists – There are menopause clinics available under the NHS, and although they are currently limited in number, your GP may refer you for specialist care when appropriate. In the private sector, there is a growing number of menopause specialists from different professional fields who may provide tailored advice and treatment. It is best to find them from a reliable source: https://thebms.org.uk/find-a-menopause-specialist/

Menopause Café support groups: https://www.menopausecafe.net/

Mobile Apps for recording and managing diet: NHS Diet Plan App; NHS Easy Meals App; NHS Food Scanner App.

Women's Health Concern: this is the patient arm of the British Menopause Society, and produces factsheets and other helpful resources - womens-health-concern.org

Appendix

The TOOLBOX – A Summary of Key Concepts, Strategies and Tools

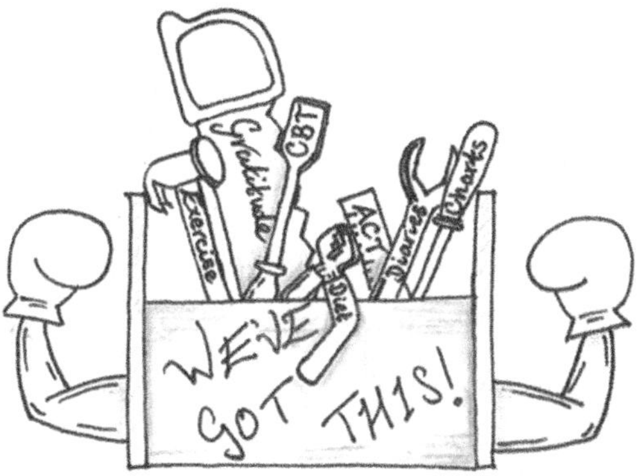

Coping with Stress, Anxiety and Worry (see Chapter 6)

Vicious cycles of anxiety

This diagram uses the CBT approach to understanding the links between our thoughts, feelings and behaviours as reactions to a situation. It shows how the way we view the experience can be unhelpful and lead to negative feelings and unhelpful behaviours such as avoidance.

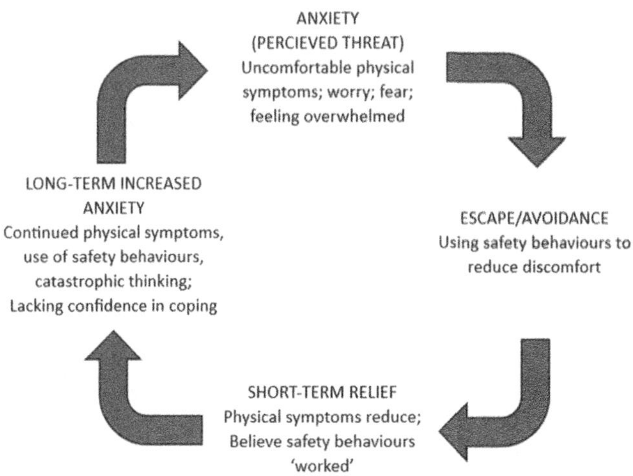

Coping cycle of anxiety

This cycle shows what it can look like when we have broken, or reversed, the vicious cycle and found a way to manage our anxiety.

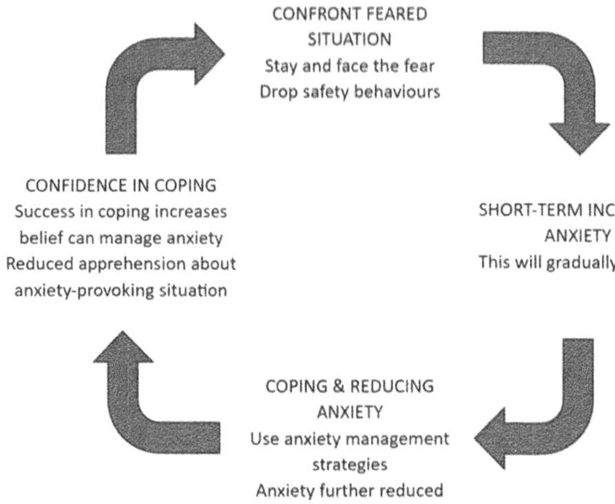

See examples of vicious cycles and coping cycles in relation to menopausal symptoms in Chapters 10, 11 and 13. Blank ones have been provided at the end of this section for your use.

Breathing exercises

Deep breathing exercises can help calm us, offsetting the physical symptoms of anxiety and prevent it escalating into panic. See the diaphragmatic breathing exercise in Chapter 6 and the square breathing exercise in Chapter 10.

Relaxation exercises

These help us cope more easily with anxiety, worry and a range of menopausal symptoms. See the progressive muscle relaxation exercise in Chapter 6 and the guided imagery meditation in Chapter 10.

Managing unhelpful thoughts and worries **(see Chapter 6)**

There are different types of techniques for challenging or relating differently to our thoughts:

- Putting things into perspective
- Thought defusion
- Thoughts on train metaphor

- Challenging unhelpful thoughts
- Setting a worry time
- Letting go of worries

Relinquishing control (see Chapter 6)

At various points in the book, we look at the concept of letting go of control and reducing our burdens to make life easier, such as these:

- Accepting that not everything is in your control
- Re-evaluating your load and shedding perfectionism
- Non-attachment

Mood Management (see Chapter 7)

'Noticing' your moods

By checking in on yourself and paying attention to your moods, you can understand them and manage them better. Practise the 'Noticing' exercise for this. You can use the weekly mood tracker at the end of this section.

Engaging in activities and with others

There are lots of things you can do to improve or maintain good mood, such as getting outdoors, engaging in activities even when you are not in the mood and connecting with others. Make sure your activities are meaningful to you – things you enjoy and aligned with your values (see below).

Reaching out and seeking help

Talk to those close to you and seek professional help when needed.

Self-compassion

Developing a practise of showing compassion and being kind to yourself just as you would be to others you care about is an important tool for looking after yourself.

Gratitude

Making a conscious habit of acknowledging and expressing appreciation on a regular basis for the good things in life, big or small, gives you a balanced perspective, improves mood and can be motivating.

Maintaining General Wellbeing (see Chapter 8)

Establishing structure and routine – Doing physical exercise and eating nutritious meals regularly, as well as having a good sleep routine (see Chapter 13), are the essential ingredients for living well at any time, particularly during the menopause transition.

Adopting a balanced lifestyle

A healthy lifestyle is a balanced lifestyle – remember the PACE acronym in this table analogy.

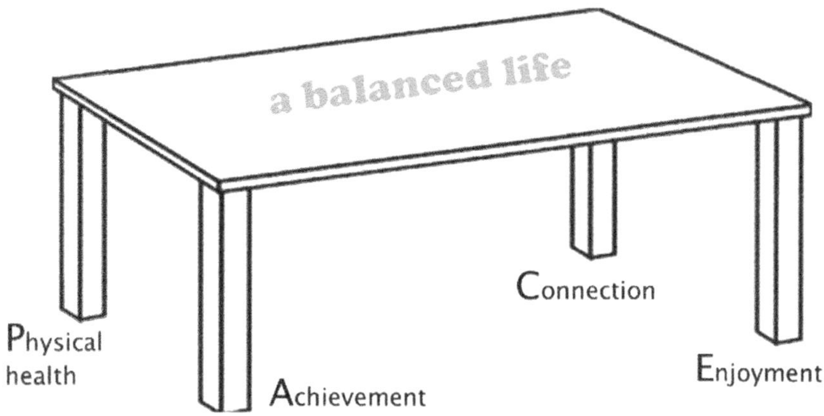

Balanced lifestyle log

Use or adapt the log provided at the end of this section to create your own structure and routine of balanced activities.

Self-care and connection

In addition to all our responsibilities, we need to give importance to caring for ourselves. Carve out some time to do what brings you joy and to connect with people whose company you enjoy and who make you feel good. And remember good communication is important for maintaining relationships.

Values, Acceptance and Spirituality (see Chapter 8)

Identifying your values

Remember there is a difference between values and goals. There are some questions you can ask yourself to identify your values; think about whether you are acting according to your values and have developed values-directed goals.

Acceptance

Practising acceptance involves allowing things to simply be – letting an experience exist without actively trying to change, deny or avoid it – and helps in dealing with challenging situations and unwanted emotions. Remember the three As of acceptance: **A**cknowledge it; **A**llow it; **A**ccommodate it.

Spirituality in action

Spiritual practices can help us cope with the stresses of life and develop a more hopeful attitude.

Problem-Solving Strategies (see Chapter 9)

Defining the problem

You might ask yourself some questions to work out what exactly the problem is. You might use the *six-step problem-solving strategy* where appropriate, or, you might use other strategies, such as these below.

Observation and recording

A practical starting point is to notice and record your thoughts, feelings and reactions to difficult situations. See the *Noticing* exercise in Chapter 7.

Tracking your menopausal symptoms

Keeping a record of your menopausal symptoms makes them feel less overwhelming and helps your own understanding, as well as providing useful information for sharing with healthcare professionals. You can use or adapt the table at the end of this section.

Goal-setting

Setting realistic goals gives you a vision of what you want to achieve. It is also motivating. To help you live a more fulfilling life and feel more grounded, make your goals meaningful to you and in line with your values (see Chapter 8). Don't forget to keep track of your progress with goals.

Mind-mapping

This helps by drawing out an overview of problem areas and your solutions as a reference point when needed (see Chapter 4).

Drawing out a vicious cycle (see **Chapter 9**)

Vicious cycles can be drawn for any problem you might feel stuck in. Fill in the blank one below for a situation you might currently be struggling with. The boxes can be filled in any order, as they are all interlinked. I suggest starting with what you notice first.

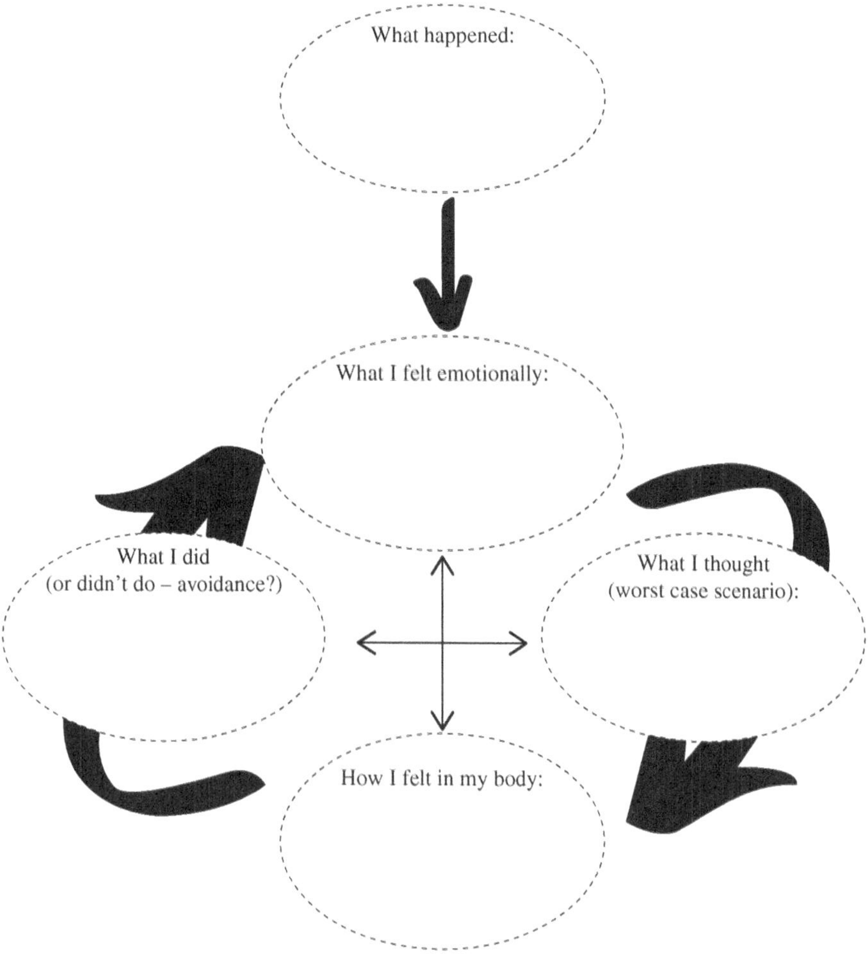

FIGURE 9.1 Vicious Cycle (blank)

Turning your vicious cycle into a coping cycle **(see Chapter 9)**

Using the coping strategies you have learnt throughout this book, and can make changes to break or reverse the vicious cycle. Draw out a coping cycle – this is a more helpful perspective, that gives you a more positive experience.

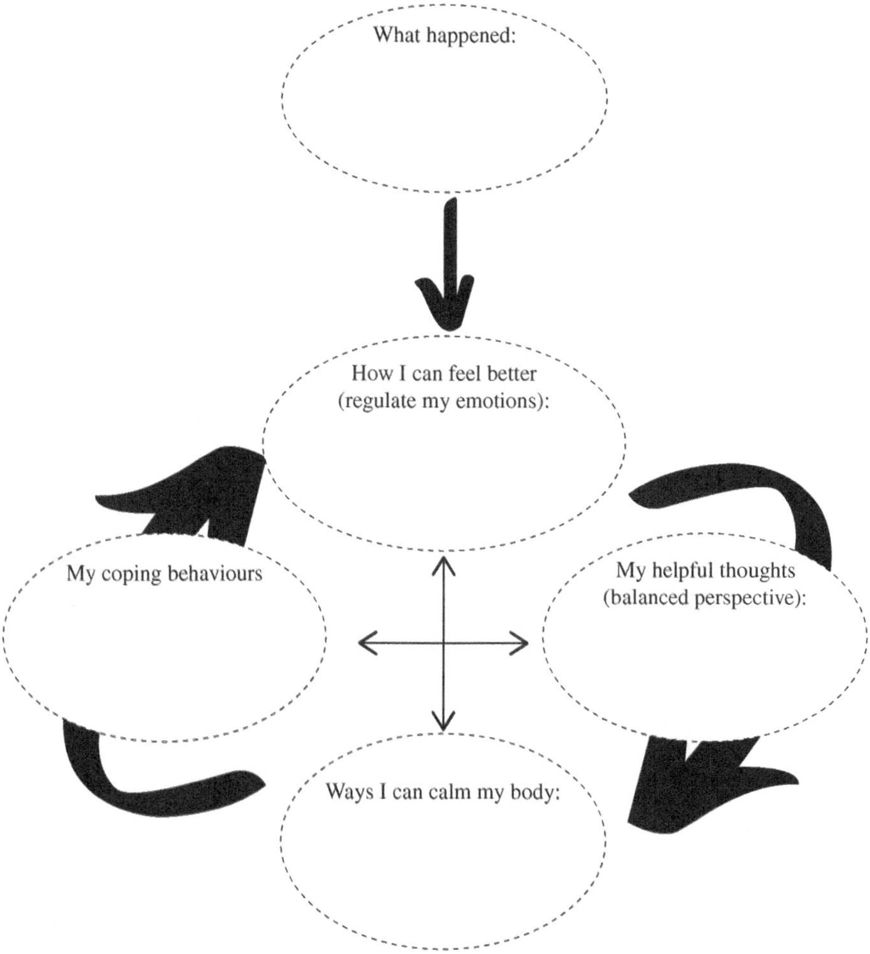

FIGURE 9.2 Coping Cycle (blank)

Weekly Mood Tracker

MOOD	Monday am	Monday pm	Tuesday am	Tuesday pm	Wednesday am	Wednesday pm	Thursday am	Thursday pm	Friday am	Friday pm	Saturday am	Saturday pm	Sunday am	Sunday pm
+3														
+2														
+1														
My normal														
-1														
-2														
-3														
Hours slept (previous night)														
Sleep quality (poor/OK/good)														
Medication														
Physical exercise														
Stressors (describe)														

In the mood section, select the box that best fits your mood rating, then in that box write a word to describe your mood. For example:

On Monday morning, if you feel worried and a little lower in mood than normal, you would write 'worried' in the -1 box for Mon am.
On Wednesday afternoon, if you're going to meet up with an old friend, you might put 'excited' in the +3 box for Wed pm.

You can give other descriptions of what's going on for you in the boxes for sleep, medication etc.

Here is a list of some words you might use to describe your mood, but of course you can use any words you want:

Happy – Calm – Excited – Pleased - Proud – Productive – Grateful – Content – Peaceful – Relaxed - Hopeful
Sad – Bored – Nervous – Angry – Irritated – Worried – Frustrated – Lonely – Stressed – Hurt – Ashamed

TABLE 7.1 Weekly Mood Tracker (see Chapter 7)

Balanced Lifestyle Log

In each time slot (can change to suit you), make a brief note of your activity. Then rate these aspects in relation to the activity on a scale of 1-10 (1=least; 10 = most): Your sense of **Achievement** for the activity on a scale of 0-10 (A=?) your sense of **Connectedness** to others/higher power (C = ?), and your sense of **Enjoyment** (E = ?) from doing the activity. At the end of each day, rate your overall mood for that day (0 = lowest to 10 = highest).

Day / Time Period	Example	Monday	Tuesday	Wednesday	Thursday	Friday	Saturday	Sunday
7 – 9 am	Got up & shower (A=4) Breakfast alone (E = 6)							
9 - 11 am	Working at home - finished report due tomorrow (A=8; E=5)							
11am-1pm	Business meeting online (A=5; C=3; E=3)							
1pm - 2pm	Prayed (C=5) Lunch (E=5) Walked to clinic (E=5)							
2 - 4pm	Two client sessions in clinic (A=9; E=7)							
4 – 6pm	Walked home; picked up shopping (A=6); Tea & 'Pointless' (E=8)(C=7)							
6 - 8pm	Online yoga (A=8; E=8); Cooked (A=8; E=7) Prayed (C=7)							
8 - 10pm	Dinner with family (C=8); Mum's call(C=6); Prepared work for tomorrow (A=7)							
10pm – 12mn	Watched TV (E=6) Prayed (C=9); Went to bed by 12 (A=9)							
MOOD RATING	8							

TABLE 8.1 Balanced Lifestyle Log (see Chapter 8)

Date/Time/Situation *Where was I when I noticed the symptom? What was I doing? What was I wearing? What time of day was it?*	**Symptom Experienced** *What did I experience? What did I notice in my body?*	**Duration/Severity** *How long did it last? How severe was it? Rate 1-10 (1= least -10 = most)*	**Emotion(s) and Thought Reaction(s)** *How did I feel when it happened? What went through my mind?*	**Behavioural Reaction(s)** *What was my immediate reaction? What helped me manage it? Did anything make it worse?*	**Other relevant information** *Could anything have triggered it? (e.g. activity/food/drink?) Was there anything else significant happening in my life at the time? (e.g. stress at work, argument with friend)*

TABLE 9.1 Menopausal Symptoms Experience Log (see Chapter 9)

Date/Time/Situation *What time of day was it? Where was I? What was I doing? Who was I with?*	**What did I eat and drink?** *List everything you ate - full meals as well as any snacks*	**Was your diet was balanced for this day? Why?/Why not?** *Think about the nutritional value of what you ate. Did you incorporate items from different food groups? You can look this up or use an app on your phone*	**Was it Emotional Eating?** *Was it a planned meal time? Was I hungry? Or was I bored, worried, anxious, upset, (or any other feeling)? Describe the feeling and rate it's intensity (0 = lowest; 10=highest)*	**Reactions and Reflections on Emotional Eating** *What might have triggered it (e.g. stress/relationship conflict)? Is there something significant happening in my life right now? Did I stop when I realised I was emotional eating? What helped me manage it? Did anything make it worse? What could I do instead of eating to cope with my feelings?*

TABLE 12.1 Food and Feelings Diary (see Chapter 12)

Sleep Diary

Complete this diary each day for one or two weeks. Complete the shaded area just before going to bed, and the non-shaded area in the morning. **For ratings: 0= least, 10 = most**

Date/Day:							
How tired I felt during the day (0-10)							
How active I was during the day (0-10)							
Time spent outside in natural light?							
My mood rating during the day (0-10)							
Any naps during the day-number/duration?							
Any exercise within 4 hours of bed?							
Caffeine, alcohol, high-sugar foods within 4 hours of bed?							
Any TV or time on phone just before bed?							
Time I went to bed?							

TABLE 13.1 Sleep Diary (see Chapter 13)

Any activity in bed – e.g. Read, TV, etc							
Time I put lights out							
Number of times I woke in the night							
Times I got out of bed-how long for?							
Time I woke up							
Total hours I slept							
Quality of sleep: I feel 0-10 (0 = exhausted; 10 = refreshed)							
Time I got out of bed							
Total hours spent in bed							
Additional notes: e.g. Stress/worry/night sweats?; sleeping pills?							

Suggestions for getting the most put of your sleep diary:

- Leave your sleep diary by your bed so you can fill it in before going to bed and when you wake up in the morning.
- Don't stress about being so accurate - an estimation of your sleep is fine, you don't have to know the exact number of times you wake us so don't try to remember it during the night as you don't want it to disrupt your sleep.
- Take a look at your daily habits (in the evening) and the quality of your sleep (in the morning) – Do you see any links between them? For example, did a behaviour such as drinking coffee or exercising too close to bedtime, lead to an outcome like poorer sleep or tiredness the next day?

TABLE 13.1 (Continued)

References

Chapter 1

1. All-Party Parliamentary Group on Menopause. Inquiry to assess the impacts of menopause and the case for policy reform. Concluding report 12th October 2022.
2. Sex, mind and the menopause (2021) Channel 4 documentary film presented by Davina McCall.
3. Singh A, Kaur S, Walia I. A historical perspective on menopause and menopausal age. *Bull Indian Inst Hist Med Hyderabad.* 2002 Jul–Dec;32(2):121–135.
4. Rudnicka E, Kruszewska J, Klicka K, et al. (2018) Premature ovarian insufficiency – aetiopathology, epidemiology, and diagnostic evaluation. *Przegląd Menopauzalny.* 2018;17:105–108.
5. Royal College of Obstetricians and Gynaecologists statement. RCOG recommends against using over-the-counter menopause tests. 10 Jun 2022. RCOG recommends against using over-the-counter menopause tests | RCOG.
6. Department of Health and Social Care. Policy paper – Women's Health Strategy for England: Details the government's 10-year ambitions and the actions we are taking now to improve the health and wellbeing of women and girls in England. Published 20 July 2022.

Chapter 2

1. NHS Website https://www.nhs.uk/conditions/periods/starting-periods/.
2. Biro FM, Greenspan LC, Galvez MP. Puberty in girls of the 21st century. *J Pediatr Adolesc Gynecol.* 2012 Oct;25(5):289–294.

Chapter 3

1. Stevenson JC, Whitehead MI. Hormone replacement therapy. *BMJ.* 2002;325:113-114.

2. Department of Health and Social Care, UK Government, NHS Hormone Replacement Therapy Prescriptions Statement UIN HCWS572 Released on 21 Feb 2023.
3. Djapardy V, Panay N. Alternative and non-hormonal treatments to symptoms of menopause. *Best Pract Res Clin Obstet Gynaecol.* 2022 May;81:45–60.
4. Shaukat A, Mujeeb A, Shahnoor S, et al. Veozah (Fezolinetant): A promising non-hormonal treatment for vasomotor symptoms in menopause. *Health Sci Rep.* 2023 Oct 5;6(10):e1610.
5. Mann E, Smith MJ, Hellier J, et al. Efficacy of a cognitive behavioural intervention to treat menopausal symptoms following breast cancer treatment (MENOS 1): A randomised controlled trial. *Lancet Oncology.* 2012;13(3):309–318.
6. Ayers B, Smith M, Hellier J, Mann E, Hunter MS. Effectiveness of group and self-help cognitive behaviour therapy to reduce problematic menopausal hot flushes and night sweats (MENOS 2): A randomized controlled trial. *Menopause.* 2012;19(7):749–759.
7. Position Statement: Non-hormonal management of menopause-associated vasomotor symptoms. The North American Menopause Society. *Menopause.* 2015;22(11):1–20.
8. BMS – Clinician's Factsheet. https://www.nice.org.uk/guidance/ng23/resources/endorsed-resource-cognitive-behaviour-therapy for-menopausal-symptoms-information-for-gps-and-health-professionals-4414178557.
9. Posadzki P, Ernst E. Prevalence of CAM use by UK climacteric women: A systematic review of surveys. *Climacteric.* 2013;16:3–7.
10. Sood R, Kuhle CL, Kapoor E, Thielen JM, Frohmader KS, Mara KC, Faubion SS. Association of mindfulness and stress with menopausal symptoms in midlife women. *Climacteric.* 2019;22(4):377–382. Published online: 17 Jan 2019.
11. Wang F, Szabo A. Effects of yoga on stress among healthy adults: A systematic review. *Altern Ther Health Med.* 2020 Jul;26(4):AT6214.
12. Woodyard C. Exploring the therapeutic effects of yoga and its ability to increase quality of life. *Int J Yoga.* 2011 Jul–Dec;4(2):49–54.
13. Cramer H, Peng W, Lauche R. Yoga for menopausal symptoms—a systematic review and meta-analysis. *Maturitas.* 2018;109:13–25.
14. National Institute for Health and Care Excellence NICE guideline NG23. Menopause: diagnosis and management, Nov 2015.

Chapter 4

1. Engel GL. The need for a new medical model: A challenge for biomedicine. *Science.* 1977;196(4286):129–136.

2. Akbari M, Hossaini SM. The relationship of spiritual health with quality of life, mental health, and burnout: The mediating role of emotional regulation. *Iran J Psychiatry.* 2018;13(1):22–31. PMID:29892314.
3. Yildirim Kurtulus H, Meral K, Kurtulus E, Kahveci H. The relationship between spirituality and psychological wellness: A serial multi-mediation analysis. *International Journal of Psychology and Educational Studies.* 2022;9(4):1160–1172.
4. Gonçalves JP, Lucchetti G, Menezes PR, Vallada H. Religious and spiritual interventions in mental health care: A systematic review and meta-analysis of randomized controlled clinical trials. *Psychol Med.* 2015;45(14):2937–2949.
5. Badri M. *Abu-Zayd al-Balkhi's 'Sustenance of the Soul: The Cognitive Behavioural Therapy of a Ninth Century Physician* (Translation & annotation). Int. Inst of Islamic Thought; 2013.
6. Beck AT, Rush AJ, Shaw BF. *Cognitive Therapy of Depression.* Guildford Press; 1979.
7. Hayes SC, Strosahl KD, Wilson KG. *Acceptance and Commitment Therapy: An Experiential Approach to Behavior Change.* Guilford Press; 1999.
8. Harris R. *ACT Made Simple*, 2nd edition. New harbinger Publications, Inc; 2019.
9. Norman J. Exploring the history of information and media through timelines. HistoryofInformation.com.
10. Buzan T, Buzan B. *The Mind Map Book.* BCA by arrangement with BBC Books; 1993.
11. Williams M, et al. Mind maps: An aid to effective formulation. *Behav. & Cogn. Psychotherapy.* 1997;25:261–267.

Chapter 5

1. The Fawcett Society. Menopause and the workplace; 2022. https://www.fawcettsociety.org.uk Accessed 01.09 2023.
2. Jaeger MB, Miná CS, Alves S, Schuh GJ, Wender MC, Manfro GG. Negative affect symptoms, anxiety sensitivity, and vasomotor symptoms during perimenopause. *Braz J Psychiatry.* 2021 May–Jun;43(3):277–284.
3. Bromberger JT, Kravitz HM, Chang Y, et al. Does risk for anxiety increase during the menopausal transition? Study of Women's Health Across the Nation. *Menopause.* 2013;20:488–495.
4. Carpenter JS, Cortés YI, Tisdale JE, Sheng Y, Jackson EA, Barinas-Mitchell E, Thurston RC. Palpitations across the menopause transition in SWAN: Trajectories, characteristics, and associations with subclinical cardiovascular disease. *Menopause.* 2023 Jan 1;30(1):18–27.
5. Marsh WK, Gershenson B, Rothschild AJ. Symptom severity of bipolar disorder during the menopausal transition. *Int J Bipolar Disord.* 2015;3:35.

6. Maki PM, Kornstein SG, Joffe H, et al. Guidelines for the evaluation and treatment of perimenopausal depression: Summary and recommendations. *Journal of Women's Health.* 2019;28:117–134.
7. Bromberger JT, Kravitz HM, Chang Y, et al. Major depression during and after the menopausal transition: Study of Women's Health Across the Nation. *Psychol Med.* 2011;41:1879–1888.
8. Bromberger JT, Schott L, Kravitz HM, Joffe H. Risk factors for major depression during midlife among a community sample of women with and without prior major depression: Are they the same or different? *Psychol Med.* 2015;45:1653–1664.
9. Schmidt PJ, Rubinow DR. Sex hormones and mood in the perimenopause. *Annals of the New York Academy of Sciences.* 2009;1179:70–85.
10. Kulkarni J. Perimenopausal depression – an under-recognised entity. *Australian Prescriber.* 2018;41:183–185.
11. Kulkarni J, Gavrilidis E, Hudaib HR, et al. Development and validation of a new rating scale for perimenopausal depression – the Meno-D. *Translational Psychiatry.* 2018a;8:123.
12. Greene J. A factor analytic study of climacteric symptoms. *Journal of Psychosomatic Research.* 1976;20:425–430.
13. National Institute for Health and Care Excellence NICE guideline NG23. Menopause: Diagnosis and management, Nov 2015.
14. Usall J, Pinto-Meza A, Fernández A, et al. Suicide ideation across reproductive life cycle of women. Results from a European epidemiological study. *Journal of Affective Disorders.* 2009;116:144–147.
15. An SY, Kim Y, Kwon R, Lim G-y, Choi HR, Namgoung S, Jeon SW, Chang Y, Ryu S. Depressive symptoms and suicidality by menopausal stages among middle-aged Korean women. *Epidemiology and Psychiatric Sciences.* 2022;31:e60, 1–8.
16. Office for National Statistics. Middle-aged generation most likely to die by suicide and drug poisoning. 2019. https://www.ons.gov.uk/peoplepopulationandcommunity/healthandsocialcare/healthandwellbeing/articles/middleagedgenerationmostlikelytodiebysuicideanddrugpoisoning/2019-08-13.
17. Independent. Fear of being labelled hysterical: 1 in 10 women experience suicidal thoughts due to perimenopause. 2021. https://www.independent.co.uk/news/uk/home-news/perimenopause-suicidal-thoughts-menopause-mental-health-b1933346.html.
18. Rekkas PV, Wilson AA, Lee VWH, et al. Greater monoamine oxidase A binding in perimenopausal age as measured with carbon 11–Labeled harmine positron emission tomography. *JAMA Psychiatry.* 2014;71(8):873–879.
19. Schulz R, Sherwood PR. Physical and mental health effects of family caregiving. *Am J Nurs.* 2008 Sep;108(9 Suppl):23–27; quiz 27.
20. Health Education England NHS, Neurodiversity Support.

21. Moseley RL, Druce T, Turner-Cobb JM. 'When my autism broke': A qualitative study spotlighting autistic voices on menopause. *Autism.* 2020;24(6):1423–1437.
22. ADDitude Expert Webinar. Menopause and ADHD: How estrogen changes impact dopamine, cognition, and women's health [Video Replay & Podcast #380] with Janette Wasserstein, Ph.D., broadcast live 18.11.21.

Chapter 6

1. Jacobson E. *Progressive Relaxation.* University of Chicago Press; 1938.
2. Morin CM, Hauri PJ, Espie CA, Spielman AJ, Buysse DJ, Bootzin RR. Nonpharmacologic treatment of chronic insomnia. An American Academy of Sleep Medicine review. *Sleep.* 1999 Dec 15;22(8):1134–1156.
3. Kabat-Zinn J. Defining mindfulness. What is mindfulness? The founder of mindfulness-based stress reduction explains. Accessed Dec 2023. https://www.mindful.org/jon-kabat-zinn
4. Khusid MA, Vythilingham M. The emerging role of mindfulness meditation as effective self-management strategy, part 1: Clinical implications for depression, post-traumatic stress disorder, and anxiety. *Military Medicine.* 2016;181(9):961–968.
5. Huang S, Wang Z, Zheng D, Liu L. Anxiety disorder in menopausal women and the intervention efficacy of mindfulness-based stress reduction. *Am J Transl Res.* 2023 Mar 15;15(3):2016–2024.
6. Gordon JL, Halleran M, Beshai S, Eisenlohr-Moul TA, Frederick J, Campbell TS. Endocrine and psychosocial moderators of mindfulness-based stress reduction for the prevention of perimenopausal depressive symptoms: A randomized controlled trial. *Psychoneuroendocrinology.* 2021;130:105277.
7. *Adapted from concept of Raisin Meditation practice in Mindfulness-Based Stress Reduction (MBSR). Developed by Jon Kabat-Zinn.
8. Wells A. *Metacognitive Therapy for Anxiety and Depression.* The Guilford Press; 2009.
9. de Botton A. *The Architecture of Happiness.* Penguin Books; 2007.

Chapter 7

1. Harris R. *ACT Made Simple,* 2nd edition: A quick-start guide to ACT basics and beyond. New Harbinger Publications, Inc; 2019.
2. Romano F, Muscogiuri G, Di Benedetto E, Zhukouskaya VV, Barrea L, Savastano S, Colao A, Di Somma C. Vitamin D and sleep regulation: Is there a role for Vitamin D? *Curr Pharm Des.* 2020;26(21):2492–2496.

3. Barton J, Pretty J. What is the best dose of nature and green exercise for improving mental health? A multi-study analysis. *Environmental Science & Technology.* 2010;44(10):3947–3955.
4. McCullough ME, Emmons RA, Tsang JA. The grateful disposition: A conceptual and empirical topography. *JPSP.* 2002;82:112–127.
5. Dickens LR. Using gratitude to promote positive change: A series of meta-analyses investigating the effectiveness of gratitude interventions. *BASP.* 2017;39:193–208.
6. Lin CC. Gratitude and depression in young adults: The mediating role of self-esteem and well-being. *Personality and Individual Differences.* 2015;87:30–34.
7. Iodice JA, Malouff JM, Schutte NS. The association between gratitude and depression: A meta-analysis. *International Journal of Depression and Anxiety.* 2021 June 23.
8. Holt-Lunstad J, Smith TB, Baker M, Harris T, Stephenson D. Loneliness and social isolation as risk factors for mortality: A meta-analytic review. *Perspect Psychol Sci.* 2015 Mar;10(2):227–237.
9. Independent. Fear of being labelled hysterical: 1 in 10 women experience suicidal thoughts due to perimenopause. 06 October 2021. Accessed Dec 2023. https://www.independent.co.uk/news/uk/home-news/perimenopause-suicidal-thoughts-menopause-mental-health-b1933346.html.

Chapter 8

1. NHS Digital. Health Survey England Additional Analyses, Ethnicity and Health, 2011-2019 Experimental statistics Fruit and vegetable consumption. Accessed Dec 2023. https://digital.nhs.uk/data-and-information/publications/statistical/health-survey-england-additional-analyses/ethnicity-and-health-2011-2019-experimental-statistics
2. World Health Organization (WHO). Website (accessed Dec 2023) Factsheet - Physical activity for adults aged 18–64 years. https://www.who.int/news-room/fact-sheets/detail/physical-activity.
3. Aknin L, Norton M, Dunn EW. From wealth to well-being? Money matters, but less than people think. *The Journal of Positive Psychology* 2009;4:6, 523–527.
4. Waldinger R, Schulz M. *The Good Life: Lessons from the World's Longest Scientific Study of Happiness.* Simon and Schuster; 2003.
5. World Health Organization (WHO). https://www.who.int/.
6. Martell CR, Addis ME, Jacobson NS. *Behavioural Activation for Depression: A Clinician's Guide.* First Edition. Guilford Press; 2013.
7. Vetrani C, Barrea L, Rispoli R, et al. Mediterranean diet: What are the consequences for menopause? *Front Endocrinol (Lausanne).* 2022 Apr 25;13:886824.

8. Grajek M, Krupa-Kotara K, Białek-Dratwa A, Sobczyk K, Grot M, Kowalski O, Staśkiewicz W. Nutrition and mental health: A review of current knowledge about the impact of diet on mental health. *Front Nutr.* 2022 Aug 22;9:943998.
9. Bożek A, Nowak PF, Blukacz M. The relationship between spirituality, health-related behavior, and psychological well-being. *Front Psychol.* 2020 Aug 14;11:1997.
10. Harris R. *ACT Made Simple (2nd Edition): A Quick-Start Guide to ACT Basics and Beyond.* New Harbinger Publications, Inc; 2019.
11. Hayes SC, Strosahl K, Wilson KG. *Acceptance and Commitment Therapy: Understanding and Treating Human Suffering.* Guilford Press; 1999.

Chapter 9

1. World Health Organization (WHO). Website (accessed Dec 2023) Factsheet - Physical activity for adults aged 18–64 years. https://www.who.int/news-room/fact-sheets/detail/physical-activity.

Chapter 10

1. British Menopause Society: BMS-Infographics-JANUARY-2023-NationalSurveyResults.pdf (thebms.org.uk).
2. Kaunitz AM, Manson JE. Management of menopausal symptoms. *Obstet Gynecol.* 2015 Oct;126(4):859–876.
3. Avis NE, Crawford SL, Greendale G, et al. Duration of menopausal vasomotor symptoms over the menopause transition. *JAMA Intern Med.* 2015 Apr;175(4):531–539.
4. Santoro N, Epperson CN, Mathews SB. Menopausal symptoms and their management. *Endocrinol Metab Clin North Am.* 2015 Sep;44(3):497–515.
5. Freeman EW, Sammel MD, Lin H, et al. The role of anxiety and hormonal changes in menopausal hot flashes, *Menopause.* 2005 May–Jun;12(3):258–266.
6. Freeman EW, Sammel MD. Anxiety as a risk factor for menopausal hot flashes: Evidence from the Penn Ovarian Aging Cohort. *Menopause.* 2016 Sep;23(9):942–949.
7. Gallicchio L, Millar SR, Kiefer J, et al. Change in body mass index, weight, and hot flashes: A longitudinal analysis from the midlife women's health study. *J Womens Health (Larchmt).* 2014 Mar 1;23(3):231–237.
8. Freedman RR. Physiology of hot flashes. *Am J Hum Biol.* 2001;13:453–464.
9. Sood R, Sood A, Wolf SL, Linquist BM, Liu H, Sloan JA, Satele DV, Loprinzi CL, Barton DL. Paced breathing compared with usual breathing for hot flashes. *Menopause.* 2013 Feb;20(2):179–184.

10. Pascoe MC, Thompson DR, Ski CK. Yoga, mindfulness-based stress reduction and stress-related physiological measures: A meta-analysis. *Psychoneuroendocrinology.* 2017;86:152–168.
11. Harris R. 2019. www.TheHappinessTrap.com.
12. Harris R. *ACT Made Simple (2nd Edition): A Quick-Start Guide to ACT Basics and Beyond.* New Harbinger Publications, Inc; 2019.

Chapter 11

1. The Fawcett Society. Menopause and the workplace; 2022. Available from: https://www.fawcettsociety.org.uk Accessed September 01, 2023.
2. Harper JC, Phillips S, Biswakarma R, Yasmin E, Saridogan E, Radhakrishnan S, C Davies M, Talaulikar V. An online survey of perimenopausal women to determine their attitudes and knowledge of the menopause. *Womens Health (Lond).* 2022 Jan–Dec;18:17455057221106890.
3. Maki PM, Springer G, Anastos K, Gustafson DR, Weber K, Vance D, Dykxhoorn D, Milam J, Adimora AA, Kassaye SG, Waldrop D, Rubin LH. Cognitive changes during the menopausal transition: A longitudinal study in women with and without HIV. *Menopause.* 2021 Jan 11;28(4):360–368.
4. Maki PM, Jaff NG. Brain fog in menopause: A health-care professional's guide for decision-making and counseling on cognition. *Climacteric.* 2022;25:570–578.
5. Epperson CN, Sammel MD, Freeman EW. Menopause effects on verbal memory: findings from a longitudinal community cohort. *J Clin Endocrinol Metab.* 2013 Sep;98(9):3829–38.
6. Mey M, Bhatta S, Casadesus G. Luteinizing hormone and the aging brain. *Vitam Horm.* 2021;115:89–104.
7. Sandi C. Memory impairments associated with stress and aging. Chapter 12 in *Neural Plasticity and Memory: From Genes to Brain Imaging.* Bermúdez-Rattoni F, editor. CRC Press/Taylor & Francis; 2007.
8. Sliwinski JR, Johnson AK, Elkins GR. Memory decline in peri- and postmenopausal women: The potential of mind-body medicine to improve cognitive performance. *Integr Med Insights.* 2014 Aug 3;9:17–23.
9. Voss MW, Vivar C, Kramer AF, van Praag H. Bridging animal and human models of exercise-induced brain plasticity. *Trends Cogn Sci.* 2013 Oct;17(10):525–544.
10. Bender CM, Sereika SM, Gentry AL, Duquette JE, Casillo FE, Marsland A, Brufsky AM, Evans S, Gorantla VC, Grahovac TL, McAuliffe PF, Steiman JG, Zhu Y, Erickson KI. Physical activity, cardiorespiratory fitness, and cognitive function in postmenopausal women with breast cancer. *Support Care Cancer.* 2021 Jul;29(7):3743–3752.

Chapter 12

1. British Menopause Society, Tool for Clinicians: Menopause: Nutrition and Weight Gain.
2. Greendale GA, Sternfeld B, Huang M, Han W, Karvonen-Gutierrez C, Ruppert K, Cauley JA, Finkelstein JS, Jiang S-F, Karlamangla AS. Changes in body composition and weight during the menopause transition. *Journal of Clinical Investigation Insight.* 2019;4(5).
3. Currie H, Moger SJ. Menopause – Understanding the impact on women and their partners. *Post Reproductive Health.* 2019;25(4):183–190.
4. Watt F. Musculoskeletal pain and menopause. *Post Reproductive Health.* 2018;24(1):34–43.
5. Magliano M. Menopausal arthralgia: Fact or fiction. *Maturitas.* 2010;67(1):29–33.
6. Ji MX, Yu Q. Primary osteoporosis in postmenopausal women. *Chronic Dis Transl Med.* 2015 Mar 21;1(1):9–13.
7. Cava E, Yeat NC, Mittendorfer B. Preserving healthy muscle during weight loss. *Adv Nutr.* 2017 May 15;8(3):511–519.
8. Figueroa A, Vicil F, Sanchez-Gonzalez MA, Wong A, Ormsbee MJ, Hooshmand S, Daggy B. Effects of diet and/or low-intensity resistance exercise training on arterial stiffness, adiposity, and lean mass in obese postmenopausal women. *Am J Hypertens.* 2013 Mar;26(3):416–423.
9. Women in Sport. Silver Linings – Understanding Women's relationship with Sportand Physical Activity in Later Life.
10. Tang Y, Liu J, Feng Z, Liu Z, Wang S, Xia Y, Geng B. Nocturnal sleep duration and bone mineral density: A cross-sectional study of the National Health and Nutrition Examination Survey (NHANES) 2007-2014. *BMC Endocr Disord.* 2022 Dec 28;22(1):333.
11. Swanson CM. Sleep disruptions and bone health: what do we know so far? *Curr Opin Endocrinol Diabetes Obes.* 2021 Aug 1;28(4):348–353.

Chapter 13

1. Russell W. *Educating Rita: A Comedy* (First ed.). Samuel French; 1981. ISBN 0-573-11115-4.
2. Currie H. Women's Health Concern Fact Sheet - Menopause and insomnia. In collaboration with the medical advisory council of the British Menopause Society; 2021.
3. Kravitz HM, Joffe H. Sleep during the perimenopause: A SWAN story. *Obstet Gynecol Clin North Am.* 2011;38:567–586.
4. *Diagnostic and Statistical Manual of Mental Disorders,* 4th edition (DSM-IV) to DSM, 5th edition (DSM-5).

5. Coborn J, de Wit A, Crawford S, Nathan M, Rahman S, Finkelstein L, Wiley A, Joffe H. Disruption of sleep continuity during the perimenopause: Associations with female reproductive hormone profiles. *J Clin Endocrinol Metab.* 2022 Sep 28;107(10):e4144–e4153.
6. Nutt D, Wilson S, Paterson L. Sleep disorders as core symptoms of depression. *Dialogues in Clinical Neuroscience.* 2008;10(3):329–336. https://pubmed.ncbi.nlm.nih.gov/18979946/.
7. NICE Guidelines for Insomnia: https://cks.nice.org.uk/topics/insomnia/management/.
8. Qaseem A, Kansagara D, Forciea M, et al. Clinical guidelines committee of the american college of P. management of chronic insomnia disorder in adults: A clinical practice guideline from the american college of physicians. *Ann Intern Med.* 2016;165(2):125–133.
9. Saldaña KS, McGowan SK, Martin JL. Acceptance and commitment therapy as an adjunct or alternative treatment to cognitive behavioral therapy for insomnia. *Sleep Med Clin.* 2023 Mar;18(1):73–83.

Chapter 14

1. Mayo Clinic Website. Ageing: What to expect aging: What to expect - Mayo Clinic; 2023.
2. Singh V, Sivakami M. Normality, freedom, and distress: Listening to the menopausal experiences of Indian women of Haryana. 2020 Jul 25. In *The Palgrave Handbook of Critical Menstruation Studies [Internet]*. Bobel C, Winkler IT, Fahs B, Hasson KA, Kissling EA, Roberts TA, editors. Singapore: Palgrave Macmillan; 2020. Chapter 70. PMID: 33347207.
3. Hoga L, Rodolpho J, Gonçalves B, Quirino B. Women's experience of menopause: A systematic review of qualitative evidence. *JBI Database System Rev Implement Rep*. 2015 Sep 16;13(8):250–337.
4. Office for National Statistics. Divorces in England and Wales: 2021 annual divorce numbers and rates, by duration of marriage, sex and to whom granted and reason. Publ 2 November 2022.
5. ''We've come a long, long way together…..' lyrics from *Praise You* by Fatboy Slim.
6. Parish SJ, Faubion SS, Weinberg M, Bernick B, Mirkin S. The MATE survey: Men's perceptions and attitudes towards menopause and their role in partners' menopausal transition. *Menopause*. 2019 Oct;26(10):1110–1116.
7. Mayo Clinic Website. Male menopause: Myth or reality? 2022. Male menopause: Myth or reality? - Mayo Clinic.
8. Office for National Statistics. ONS Birth characteristics in England and Wales: 2021. 2021.

9. Menopause Support Website (Posted on July 4, 2019) An Important Victory: Menopause will now be taught in UK secondary schools An Important Victory: Menopause will now be taught in UK secondary schools – menopausesupport.co.uk

Chapter 15

1. Office for National Statistics. Labour Market Statistics. London: Office for National Statistics. Dec 2023 Available from: https://www.ons.gov.uk/employmentandlabourmarket/peopleinwork/employmentandemployeetypes/bulletins/uklabourmarket/december2023.
2. State Pension Age Review 2023. Department of Works and Pensions, UK Govt. ISBN 978-1-5286-3730-5. ID E02808976 03/23.
3. House of Commons Women and Equalities Committee - Menopause and the workplace survey results Fourth Special Report of Session 2021–22. 23 February 2022.
4. The Fawcett Society. Menopause and the workplace; 2022. Available from: https://www.fawcettsociety.org.uk Accessed September 01, 2023.
5. Circle In - Driving the change: Menopause and the workplace – Research paper Published 30 March, 2021.
6. British Menopause Society Factsheet (2020)- Woman's relationship with the menopause is complicated…
7. Hardy C, Griffiths A, Thorne E, Hunter M. Tackling the taboo in the UK: Talking about menopause-related problems at work. *International Journal of Workplace Health Management* 2019.
8. British Standards Institute Menstrual and menopausal health matters in your workplace. BS 30416:2023 ISBN 978 0 539 23778 8 Publisher.
9. Advisory, Conciliation and Arbitration Service, ACAS. Menopause and the workplace – ACAS's response to the House of Commons Women and Equalities Select Committee's inquiry into menopause and the workplace, 2021.
10. Menopause in the Workplace Limited, in partnership with the University of Warwick have produced a '5-minute guide: Talking to your manager about menopause'.
11. Hardy C, Griffiths A, Norton S, Hunter MS. Self-help cognitive behavior therapy for working women with problematic hot flushes and night sweats (MENOS@Work): A multicenter randomized controlled trial. *Menopause.* 2018 May;25(5):508–519.
12. Department of Work and Pensions, UK Govt Policy paper *No Time to Step Back: the government's Menopause Employment Champion.* Published 18 October 2023.

Chapter 16

1. El Khoudary SR, Greendale G, Crawford SL, et al. The menopause transition and women's health at midlife: A progress report from the Study of Women's Health Across the Nation (SWAN). *Menopause.* 2019;26(10):1213–1227.
2. MacLellan J, Dixon S, Bi S, Toye F, McNiven A. Perimenopause and/or menopause help-seeking among women from ethnic minorities: A qualitative study of primary care practitioners' experiences. *British Journal of General Practice.* 2023;73(732):e511–e518.
3. Im EO, Hu Y, Cheng CY, Ko Y, Chee E, Chee W. Racial/Ethnic differences in cognitive symptoms during the menopausal transition. *West J Nurs Res.* 2019 Feb;41(2):217–237.
4. Kriplani A, Banerjee K. An overview of age of onset of menopause in northern India. *Maturitas.* 2005;52(3-4):199–204.
5. Pitkin J. Cultural issues and the menopause. *Menopause International.* 2010;16(4):156–161.
6. Qazi RA. Age, pattern of menopause, climacteric symptoms and associated problems among urban population of Hyderabad, Pakistan. *J Coll Physicians Surg Pak.* 2006 Nov;16(11):700–703.
7. Sibli S, Islam S, Uddin MJ, et al. Analysis of the average menopause age of Bangladeshi women: A public health perspective. *World Journal of Advanced Research and Reviews.* 2022;16(3):231–235.
8. Lumsden MA. Menopausal symptoms in Bangladeshi women in midlife. *Menopause.* 2016;23(7):706–707.
9. Thurston RC, Bromberger JT, Joffe H, Avis NE, Hess R, Crandall CJ, Chang Y, Green R, Matthews KA. Beyond frequency: Who is most bothered by vasomotor symptoms? *Menopause.* 2008 Sep–Oct;15(5):841–847.
10. Wang M. Age at natural menopause and associated factors in adult women: Findings from the China Kadoorie Biobank study in Zhejiang rural area. *PLoS One.* 2018;13(4).
11. Gold EB. The timing of the age at which natural menopause occurs. *Obstet Gynecol Clin North Am.* 2011 Sep;38(3):425–440.
12. Marsh EE, Shaw ND, Klingman KM, Tiamfook-Morgan TO, Yialamas MA, Sluss PM, Hall JE. Estrogen levels are higher across the menstrual cycle in African–American women compared with Caucasian women. *J Clin Endocrinol Metab.* 2011;96(10):3199–3206.
13. Richardson LJ, Goodwin AN, Hummer RA. Social status differences in allostatic load among young adults in the United States. *SSM Popul Health.* 2021;15:100771.
14. Vauclair CM, Hanke K, Huang LL, Abrams D. Are Asian cultures really less ageist than Western ones? It depends on the questions asked. *Int J Psychol.* 2017 Apr;52(2):136–144.

15. Alexander RD. The evolution of social behaviour. *Annu Rev Ecol Syst.* 1974;5:325–383.
16. Chibanda D, Weiss HA, Verhey R, et al. Effect of a primary care–based psychological intervention on symptoms of common mental disorders in Zimbabwe: A randomized clinical trial. *JAMA*. 2016;316(24):2618–2626.
17. Jones EK, Jurgenson JR, Katzenellenbogen JM, Thompson SC. Menopause and the influence of culture: Another gap for Indigenous Australian women? *BMC Womens Health*. 2012 Dec 12;12:43.
18. Mahady GB, Locklear TD, Doyle BJ, Huang Y, Perez AL, Caceres A. Menopause, a universal female experience: Lessons from Mexico and Central America. *Current Women`s Health Reviews.* 2008;4(1):3–8.
19. Singh V, Sivakami M. Normality, freedom, and distress: Listening to the menopausal experiences of Indian women of Haryana, Chapter 70 in *The Palgrave Handbook of Critical Menstruation Studies* Published online; 2020.
20. Murphy MM, Verjee MA, Bener A, Gerber LM. The hopeless age? A qualitative exploration of the experience of menopause in Arab women in Qatar. *Climacteric*. 2013 Oct;16(5):550–554.
21. Im E-O, Hee Lee S, Chee W. Sub-ethnic differences in the menopausal symptom experience: Asian American Midlife Women. *J Transcult Nurs.* 2010 Apr;21(2):123–133.
22. Genazzani AR, Schneider HP, Panay N, Nijland EA. The European Menopause Survey 2005: Women's perceptions on the menopause and postmenopausal hormone therapy. *Gynecological Endocrinology*. 2006 Jan 1;22(7):369–375.
23. Rapaport L. Culture may influence how women experience menopause. *Reuters*. (2015, June 5). Retrieved September 27, 2021, from https://www.reuters.com/article/us-health-menopause-perceptions/culture-may-influence-how-women-experience-menopause-idUSKBN0OL1XH20150605
24. Neha Bhayana Menopause: The 'ladies problem' that is no longer a taboo to Article in Times of India, Mar 26, 2023. https://timesofindia.indiatimes.com/india/menopause-the-ladies-problem-that-is-no-longer-a-taboo-topic/articleshow/99005284.cms?from=mdr.
25. Shorey S, Esperanza D. The experiences and needs of Asian women experiencing menopausal symptoms: A meta-synthesis. *Menopause*. 2019;26(5):557–569.
26. Liu J, Eden J. Experience and attitudes toward menopause in Chinese women living in Sydney - A cross sectional survey. *Maturitas.* January 2008;58(4):359–365.
27. Gupta P, Sturdee DW, Hunter MS. Mid-age health in women from the Indian subcontinent (MAHWIS): General health and the experience of menopause in women. Climacteric. 2006 Feb;9(1):13–22.

28. Harlow SD, Burnett-Bowie SAM, Greendale GA, et al. Disparities in reproductive aging and midlife health between Black and White women: The Study of Women's Health Across the Nation (SWAN). *Womens Midlife Health.* 2022;8:3.
29. inews online - *Ethnic Minority Women in England Far Less Likely to Get Menopause Treatment, Data Shows.* https://inews.co.uk/news/ethnic-minority-women-england-menopause-treatment-2201112.
30. British Menopause Society Tool for clinicians (June 2023) Menopause in ethnic minority women.
31. Richard-Davis G, Wellons M. Racial and ethnic differences in the physiology and clinical symptoms of menopause, 2013. *Seminars in Reproductive Medicine.* 2013;31(5):380–386.

Chapter 17

Hickey M, Hunter MS, Santoro N, Ussher J. Normalising menopause. *BMJ.* 2022 Jun 15;377:e069369.

About the Author

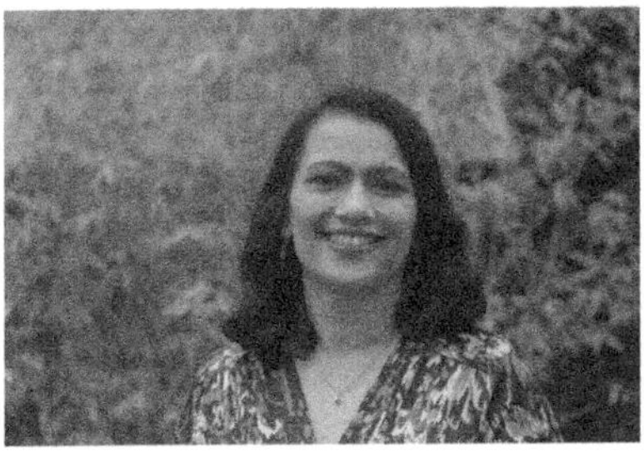

Dr Momotaj Gafur Islam is a chartered clinical psychologist, qualified in the UK, trained in a number of therapeutic approaches including CBT and ACT, and has 24 years of experience working in the National Health Service, academic institutions and private practice. She has expertise in working with adults with a range of difficulties having spent most of her career working within community mental health teams based in numerous psychiatric hospitals in London. Momotaj is bilingual and provides therapy in English and Bengali. She provides supervision to other therapists and consultancy services to charities and other organisations. She serves as chief psychologist at a company that develops digital healthcare in the mental health field.

Momotaj has always been passionate about women's issues, as well as giving back to the community. She was a trustee for a mental health charity and currently serves as a consultant for a charity setting up culturally specific services. For many years, she has been promoting mental health awareness, including making appearances on local television aimed at reducing the stigma of mental illness persistent in most communities. Her work was recognised by the Asian Women of Achievement Awards in 2017, where she was nominated and shortlisted in the Professionals category.

Printed and bound by CPI Group (UK) Ltd, Croydon, CR0 4YY
09/04/2026
02087011-0010